Healing Your Heart without Drugs or Surgery:

Creating New Arteries with EECP

ROBERT S. RISTER

This book is written from the author's personal experiences and does not constitute medical advice. Always seek and follow a licensed physician's advice for medical concerns.

Amazon Kindle Edition

Author website: www.myeecp.com

Library of Congress Cataloging-in-Publication Data

Rister, Robert S., 1955-

Healing you heart without drugs or surgery: Creating new arteries with EECP/ Robert S. Rister

1. Enhanced external counterpulsation—Popular works. 2. Heart disease—Alternative treatment—Popular works. 3. Coronary heart disease—Alternative Treatment—Popular Works I. Title

RC684.E53B73.2017

616I'—dc22

ISBN: 978-1-98042-1221

Independently published

Country of first publication: United States of America

DEDICATION

To cardiologist Dr. Ed Lefeber, whose friendship was heartening in a very hard time.

CONTENTS

HOW TO USE THIS BOOK

This book describes an extraordinary drug-free non-surgical method of cardiovascular rehabilitation called enhanced external counterpulsation, or EECP. In the preface of this book, I discuss how I finally found EECP—and how I know it worked—after eight stent procedures. In the introduction of this book, I recount the documented testimonies of others who have been treated with EECP and come from disability back to health.

Then in seven chapters I discuss what EECP is, how it works, what it does for heart health, some surprising benefits for other health concerns, who can have EECP, who can't have EECP, how to pay for EECP and what to expect in treatment, and how to maintain your gains after treatment. There are also answers to frequently asked questions, a list of scientific references for key facts in the text, a list of providers of EECP in the United States, and a glossary.

This book is a patient perspective on EECP. It is not medical advice. Your cardiologist is always your first, last, and best guidance for cardiovascular health. I hope you will find this book a source of the right questions to ask your doctor, and a guide to some of the practical aspects of EECP that you are not likely to find anywhere else. Your comments and questions are welcome on my website, myeecp.com.

PREFACE

By the time you have had seven percutaneous coronary interventions, eight angioplasties, and eight stents, you may decide "Enough is enough." At least I did. My decision was about eight years coming.

In 2009, I had a heart attack.

In 2012, I had another heart attack. And a second. And a third and a fourth and a fifth. Over a period of eight years from 2009 to 2017 I had at least 11 heart attacks. I have to stop and think to remember what happened when. My doctors have told me that they find my history challenging to follow. Probably you will, too, but I am less concerned that you can follow what happened when so much as you reach the happy ending to my story.

It was several years before I was referred to a hematologist who determined that I had a blood clotting disorder (too much clotting, not too little) that was the basic problem. It took another couple of years to find a way to treat the clotting problem. By that time I had had seven rounds of percutaneous coronary intervention, that is, angioplasty and stenting, and eight stents.

I got two stents during my first procedure. Then the doctor gave me a third stent in a second procedure. That's when disaster struck.

The second stent from the first procedure clotted off a couple of hours after I got a third stent in the second stent procedure. Both ends of the problem stent were blocked by blood clots. It had been in place about a month. I had been getting the latest and greatest blood thinner to prevent this from happening, but doctors did not know that it didn't work for about 1 percent of the population. My undiagnosed coagulation disorder but me in that 1 percent.

I went into cardiac arrest. Sudden death. Fortunately for me this happened while I was on a cardiac monitor. At that exact moment three nurses were coming into my room for three different reasons. A heart surgeon was walking down the hall by my room on rounds. An OR was vacant.

I came back to life about twelve minutes later as the doctor was saying "360, no detectible pulse." I wanted to say, "Don't send me to the morgue yet." I only managed to open my eyes. Probably the EKG told my story better than I could.

The doctor apologized that there was no time to give me an anesthetic. I felt a sharp cut. Then the doctor started something called internal counterpulsation therapy.

I also got a fourth stent in a third stent procedure just four hours after I got that third stent in my second stent procedure. The doctors kept me in the ICU for the next two days. My incisions were just packed, not sealed. This was so I could get a fifth stent in a fourth procedure, the third in three days.

By the end of that week I had a stent inside a stent where the clotting had occurred. Those were not to be my last stents. Those were not even to be my last stents in the same segment of the same artery.

I felt more or less OK for about a year. Then I started having chest pain again. I felt my heart fluttering in my chest. I was tired all the time. Every I sat down I wanted to fall asleep.

I went to see another cardiologist who told me my EKG showed something called supraventricular tachyarrhythmias, or SVTs. I didn't have atrial fibrillation, A-fib, but I was feeling awful. The cardiologist scheduled me for another percutaneous coronary intervention. It was back to the cath lab for me.

The cardiologist found that the artery that had been opened by angioplasty and stents twice was 80 percent closed again. I had a "balloon" (a pseudoaneurysm) in the artery where blood was backed up. My surgeon turned the screen around so I could watch the "balloon" deflate and blood flow return to normal as he placed yet another stent. This stent left my RCA "broadly patent," the doctor said, freely flowing.

But at this point I had more than a "full metal jacket." September 2012 my interventionist had placed a 14 mm stent in the proximal (nearest to the heart) segment of my right coronary artery (RCA). In October 2012 he placed a 15 mm stent inside the 14 mm stent in the same segment of my RCA. On this next trip to the catheterization lab, in August of 2014, another interventionist placed a 16 mm stent inside the 15 mm stent inside the 14 mm stent in that part of my RCA. That third stent left my RCA "broadly patent," the doctor said, blood flowing freely.

I felt great after the procedure for a while, but the results were not to last forever. Late in 2016 I started feeling lousy again. In February of 2017 after intervening in a fight between two neighbors at two o'clock in the morning I had my eleventh heart attack. I was rushed to the ER, and sent to the catheterization lab yet again.

The segment of the artery one doctor had opened in 2014 was now "100 percent closed" again. I got a fourth stent in the same location, a 15 mm stent inside a 16 mm stent inside a 15 mm stent inside a 14 mm stent. If the stents had not been made of copper and platinum, I would probably set off metal detectors. Once again, the artery was flowing freely after the procedure. But this was the fourth time around for the same procedure.

I asked what could be done if this stent failed, too. "We'll give you another one," the doctor said. Then I asked another question. "Wait a minute. If my RCA was 100 percent blocked, how was I alive and functional before I had the heart attack?"

In 2015 my cardiologist had referred me for a treatment called enhanced external counterpulsation therapy, or EECP. It's designed to encourage the heart to create collateral circulation. Collateral circulation is a kind of natural bypass. I had had just 10 treatments before another health concern intervened. But in just 10 treatments my heart had grown a collateral artery around the blockage sending blood where it needed to go.

When my doctor told me he was referring me to EECP and some of the astounding results it had had for his other patients, my reaction was something on the lines of "Yeah, right." But just a couple of weeks of treatment apparently had left me with an entirely new blood vessel. This was an entirely new blood vessel that was keeping me alive. It was doing what stents could not.

So I decided that rather than go for a stent inside a stent inside a stent inside a stent inside a stent the next time

I had heart pain, maybe it was time to try something new. After all, doing less than half the prescribed treatment had produced the desired result.

I would hardly be the first person who opted for EECP over further surgical intervention. There are many people who can tell you that EECP works. In the Introduction I will recount some of their stories.

INTRODUCTION

Hundreds of thousands of people around the world have chosen the heart treatment EECP. For reasons that will be clear as we go along, I like to call it "getting pumped." Throughout this book I will refer to my own experiences, but I would like to start with six testimonials you can verify for yourself.

Dr. Robert Turner was a superintendent of education who came to known as the "father of gifted education in Virginia." He was diagnosed with heart disease in 1972 at the age of 49. Over the next 20 years he underwent "more catheterizations than I can count." He had a series of angioplasties.

The longest the relief from any angioplasty lasted for Dr. Turner was just three weeks. He held up through a failed first and second bypass operation, and then the doctor told him he needed a third. The doctor told him he only had a 40 percent chance of surviving the procedure. "I don't like to have my patients die on the table," the doctor said.

At the age of 69, Dr. Turner wasn't ready to call it quits. Researching his alternatives, he found enhanced external counterpulsation therapy, a treatment more commonly known as EECP. He got the 35 standard treatments. "My life wasn't worth living before EECP," Dr. Turner said, but after the treatments he was able to manage a timber farm and a cattle operation. Six years after getting pumped up with EECP Dr. Turner said, "I'll admit that a few times a year I get chest pains when I have to chase the cows." But before EECP, he was bedridden.[1]

(Throughout this introduction and the next seven chapters I will have endnotes for citations of sources. They are organized by chapter in the section Endnotes after Frequently Asked Questions.)

Molly missed being able to cook Sunday dinner after church for her 17 family members plus several neighbors. She would start the meal, but she found herself so out of breath she would have to lie down. Eventually, Molly had to give up family dinners altogether. Then her doctor gave her a referral to EECP. After Molly's first week of treatment, her youngest granddaughter told her how much she missed seeing her grandma every Sunday, so Molly promised to make the meal the very next Sunday. Molly cooked for 19 people with ease, and even took charge of cleaning up the kitchen afterward.

Molly told her EECP provider Legacy Heart Care: "After a couple weeks of receiving EECP® treatments I had an appointment to see my physician, he was so impressed. He couldn't believe how much easier I was breathing and the increased amount of energy was obvious. He immediately turned to a young physician in his internship and told him to take this material back to his professors because everybody needs to know about EECP."[2]

Seventy-six year-old Justine Reynolds of Centerburg, Ohio went to see a cardiologist after repeated episodes of an odd sensation something like feeling a sponge soaking up water in the middle of her chest. After a thallium stress test and angiography, Justine got the news that she had blockages in three coronary arteries, one of which was 99 percent closed. The doctor offered her a choice between bypass surgery and EECP.

Justine asked several friends who were nurses for advice, and settled on going forward with EECP. Her friends also accompanied her to treatment. They were afraid that the pressure cuffs would be too much for her. " "It's true that you can't help noticing the air pressure, but it's nothing to shy away from. In fact, I miss that thing. Maybe I need to be shook up," said Justine. A year after treatment Justine was once again able to mow her own lawn with a push-mower, something she had not been able to do in several years.

Justine rejoined her walking group. She was able to volunteer for Interchurch Social Services and attend several meetings each month. At one meeting, a gentleman also volunteering remarked that her color was a lot better than it used to be. "You know there's a real change if a man can notice a difference," said Justine.[3]

Dr. Julian Whitaker tells the story of his patient Chester. Chester had angina pain so severe that walking just 20 steps brought on unbearable chest pain. The cardiologist ordered an angiogram. Four blocked arteries were found. He was sent to the ICU to await bypass surgery, but decided to check himself out against medical advice.

Chester then consulted Dr. Whitaker, who recommended 35 treatments with EECP. At the end of the seven weeks of treatment, Chester was able to walk a mile and a half twice a day without pain.[4]

Dr. Whitaker says that Chester's story is "more dramatic than most," but it fits the pattern or relief from shortness of breath and angina without surgical intervention, without chelation therapy, and without prescription medications.

Not everyone who uses EECP has heart disease. Famous quarterback Payton Manning got such good results from EECP he was accused of using human growth hormone.[5] EECP was also part of basketball great Shaquille O'Neal's workout regimen when he was still playing.[6] It has also been used by the Chinese military to improve fitness of soldiers.[7]

These are just a few of tens of thousands of personal stories about the effectiveness of EECP, but not all the testimonials for EECP are purely anecdotal. They also appear in peer-reviewed medical literature.

CHAPTER 1. WHAT IS EECP?

EECP, which is short for "enhanced external conterpulsation therapy," is a non-surgical, no-drugs method of growing new blood vessels. Over a period of seven weeks patients are treated with passive exercise. By "passive" I mean that the EECP equipment does the workout for you, but your body still benefits.

At the beginning of every EECP session, technicians attach something that looks like oversized blood pressure cuffs to the legs and abdomen. The cuffs inflate every time the heart rests, and deflate every time the heart beats. This counter rhythm to the heart creates a counter flow of blood back to the heart that oxygenates and nourishes it. The backwards flow of blood also sets off a series of hormonal reactions that trigger a process called angiogenesis, the grown of new blood vessels. After six or seven weeks, or even sooner, the heart creates new coronary arteries. There also can be new blood vessels elsewhere in the body. EECP confers the benefits of working out hard for years, but these benefits are realized in less than two months.

The key to understanding EECP. There is one thing you need to know to understand EECP: Arteries aren't pipes. When a pipe gets clogged, flow through it stops. That flow will back up to its source, and if water keeps flowing in, eventually a gasket is going to blow somewhere.

Arteries are different in a very important way. When an artery gets clogged, blood flows back, too, but the human body is a living organism. The vessels that sent blood toward the clog can constrict and increase pressure. This helps blood flow past the clog. And if blood flows backwards often enough, the circulatory system can slowly remodel itself so blood bypasses the area of occlusion. Pipes can't do their own plumbing. Arteries can. The new plumbing the body creates when there is backflow of blood is called a collateral artery.

Collateral arteries take over when original arteries fail. When I had my first heart attack, my left anterior descending artery (LAD) was 100 percent blocked. My right coronary artery (RCA) was over 80 percent blocked. However, I had walked into the hospital despite having very little flow through these two vital coronary arteries. How was this possible?

Over the years that my LAD and RCA had been closed off by atherosclerosis, my heart had managed to grow two new arteries to send blood around the areas of vascular injury. Fortunately, I had exercised an hour or two a day for over 30 years. When I exercised, blood flowed backward around hardened, growing, calcified cholesterol plaques. But a hormonal reaction in the heart had sustained the growth of two collateral arteries to replace the two closed arteries.

EECP seemed to be too good to be true for me, but it actually worked. Collateral arteries can be "good as new." Or they can be large enough to prevent death but not large enough to support normal activity. My collaterals were in that second category. They kept me from dying (or even feeling particularly sick) during a widowmaker heart attack, but they weren't enough for me to pursue ordinary activities outside a hospital bed. I needed treatment. The option available to me was at the time was stenting.

However, after receiving seven stents in six procedures over three years, when I had angina pain yet again, my cardiologist suggested something different. He sent me to a center that does EECP. Frankly, I was skeptical.

The nurse practitioner I saw at the center made a hard sell to convince me of the seemingly too simple idea of EECP: If you can increase the backward flow into coronary (and other) arteries to accelerate the growth of new collaterals. Instead of growing a collateral artery over, say, seven years, with EECP it is possible to grow multiple collaterals in just seven weeks. There's no surgery. There's no medication. You don't have to change your diet or exercise. You just need to go through a series of treatments I call "getting pumped." Getting pumped is all you need, or at least the staff of the center assured me that it was. A good standard of medical care, getting the right medications to stabilize blood pressure and heart rhythm, and treating cholesterol and inflammation, are still essential even if you get EECP. But EECP, it turns out, can do most of the things percutaneous coronary intervention (angioplasty and stents) can do. It just takes a little longer to do them.

What do I mean by getting pumped? In EECP, the patient is placed on a bed next to an EKG monitor. A device that looks something like a giant blood pressure cuff is attached to the lower legs, and the thighs, and the abdomen. The cuffs inflate and deflate in rhythm with the patient's heartbeat. During systole, when the heart pushes oxygenated blood out, the cuffs deflate. During diastole, when the heart is resting between beats, the cuffs inflate and send blood backward through the arteries.

What does sending blood backward do? It triggers the release of angiogenic growth factors that stimulate the creation of new blood vessels. But the size and pressure of the device causes the release of high concentrations of these growth factors.

In just 10 sessions in 2015, I would discover in 2017, EECP had caused my heart to create a collateral vessel that had not been there before. Years and years of working out two hours a day had given me two collateral vessels that probably saved my life as atherosclerosis destroyed the blood vessels I had been born with. What a catheterization showed in 2017 that a catheterization did not show in 2015 was a new artery across the lower half of my heart. Even though I had a 100 percent blockage of the right coronary artery, I was more or less functional until I had to deal with violent neighbors at two o'clock one morning. Right up to that heart attack, the new artery that appeared after just 10 EECP sessions had compensated for the stent inside the stent inside the stent that had failed a third time. I only discovered the third stent had failed, too, by having yet another mild heart attack during an especially emotional confrontation leading up to my calling the police.

Yes, I did have another heart attack. But despite the fact my RCA was 100 percent closed—again—after not one, not two, but three stents in the same location, I had been going about my life without a functioning RCA. I had functioning collateral, which was enough. And I had it thanks to EECP. But how does EECP change the circulatory system?

For those of you who are wondering why I had just 10 EECP treatments in 2015, the explanation is to be found in our Memorial Day floods of that year. I had to wade through sewage-tainted flood waters. I had tiny, pinprick-sized cut on my big toe. That tiny cut was big enough to let in a variety of toxic bacteria that caused me to have sepsis and septic shock a few weeks later. I had to interrupt EECP to spend 52 days in hospital dealing with sepsis. That kind of infection, by the way, is a contraindication for EECP that isn't often discussed. I'll discuss it the Frequently Asked Questions chapter later in this book.

CHAPTER 2. HOW EECP WORKS

To understand how EECP works, I have noted before, it is first necessary to put aside some common but outdated ideas about the circulatory system.

Human blood vessels aren't "pipes." They are living organs. They are elastic. They can, within limits, shrink and expand. This is how they maintain optimal blood pressure for optimal blood flow.

You really don't want flexible plumbing in your house. You want your house's pipes to deliver the same flow all the time. But you do want flexible "plumbing" in your body. Your body is not an inanimate object. Sometimes your body needs more blood flow. Sometimes it needs less. Stiff arteries are as big a problem as blocked arteries. But collateral arteries can compensate for both problems. EECP stimulates your body to build collateral arteries.

Collateral arteries are activated by changes in pressure. These tiny potential arteries in the heart (and elsewhere in the body) remain in a state of hibernation until they are activated by a change in the pressure gradient around them. A blockage in artery results in higher pressure on the closer-to-the-heart side of the blockage and lower pressure on the farther-from-the-heart side of the blockage.

As the blockage grows and the difference between the two pressures increases, angiogenic growth factors cause the collateral blood vessels to grow and mature. Angiogenic growth factors, you may recall from Chapter 1, are the substances that trigger the growth of new blood vessels. The maximum production of these growth factors occurs when the pressure gradient increases to the point that the flow of blood is reversed around the blockage.

The greater the pressure, the greater the growth of new blood vessels. EECP concentrates pressure just enough to maximize growth of new channels for blood flow. EECP, as we covered earlier, reverses the flow of blood through collaterals. Just one hour of EECP can result in 21 percent increase in the release of a protein called VEGF (vascular endothelial growth factor) —for the next month.

The greater the stress on a collateral vessel, the more it will grow. The longer the stress on a collateral vessel, the more it will grow. Collateral vessels will continue to grow until the heart can pump the greatest possible volume of blood with the least possible effort.

EECP also reduces inflammation and stimulates the production of "NO." EECP doesn't just cause blood vessels to grow. It also reduces inflammation. By reducing inflammation, the increased blood flow during EECP fights a fundamental cause of atherosclerosis.

And the new blood vessels the body creates in response to EECP are more flexible. They are more capable of expanding to lower pressure and tightening to raise it. Treatment with EECP enables to produce less of the chemical endothelin (ET-1) and more of the chemical nitric oxide (NO).

What are ET-1 and NO?

ET-1 causes the endothelium, the protective layer around blood vessels to constrict. This tension increases blood pressure. The heart has to work harder to pump blood against the vascular resistance triggered by ET-1.

ET-1 also increases the production of two hormones, aldosterone and atrial natriuretic peptide. These hormones force the body to retain sodium and water. Congestive heart failure may result.

While ET-1 is harmful, NO is helpful. Nitric oxide makes the lining of arteries less susceptible to clots, cracks, and spasms, which protects the circulatory system from the ravages of congestive heart failure, diabetes, high blood pressure, high cholesterol, obesity, and vascular injury.

One study found that EECP reduces the production of ET-1 by 32 to 48 percent during treatment. That's why many EECP patients suddenly begin to lose water weight about the middle of their programs. ET-1 reduction is still about 10 percent even three months after the treatment is over.

That same study found that EECP increases production of NO by 45 to 79 percent during treatment, and NO levels were still 1 to 23 percent higher three months after completion of treatment.[1]

There have been hundreds of studies of EECP from its inception over 60 years ago. I'll highlight just a few.

EECP is a non-surgical way to accomplish the same things as an earlier surgical technique. I have found that some people need to understand how EECP came into being to be comfortable having it. I am including a very brief history of the scientific development of EECP here. But if you aren't interested in the history of the technique, please feel free to skip down to the next section on the results of clinical testing.

In 1953 Dr. Adrian Kantrowitz, then at Harvard Medical School, described a method of "diastolic augmentation" to improve blood flow to the heart. By the early 1960's Kantrowitz and his research team at Grace-Sinai Hospital in Detroit had developed a device for *internal* counterpulsation therapy for treatment of cardiogenic shock. (That's what I had after a cardiac arrest.)

The surgeon would open the femoral artery, the same artery that is accessed for most modern stent procedures. Then the surgeon would thread a catheter through the artery to a site in the aorta about 2 cm (a little less than an inch) from the left subclavian artery. The balloon was designed to inflate between heart beats (diastole) and deflate during heart beats (systole). The inflated balloon would create a slight vacuum that drew blood back to the heart with each beat. This decreased the oxygen demand of the heart at the same time it increased the oxygen supply to the heart. The balloons for *internal* counterpulsation therapy became commercially available in 1967.

While several research teams were working on internal counterpulsation therapy, Dr. W. C. Birtwell and his colleagues at Harvard Medical School were developing a device for *external, non-surgical* counterpulsation therapy. They created a set of cuffs applied to the legs that were inflated and deflated by the flow of water, instead of air. This early EECP setup was bulky and hard to use, but it had a major advantages of internal counterpulsation therapy. Surgery was not necessary. And not only did the device increase blood flow to the heart, it increased venous return all over the body.[2]

Both of these devices increased survival rates for people who had had heart attacks. Both devices reduced angina. But about this time the attention of the medical world was captured by two new techniques, angioplasty and bypass surgery. These newer techniques that produced dramatic results (and generated vastly higher revenues for hospitals and doctors) captured the attention of cardiologists.

Even so, some doctors continued to refine the technique. In the 1970's, engineers had designed a set of cuffs that were inflated with air rather than with water and that inflated sequentially rather than all at the same time. This refinement of technique made EECP much easier to use.

And by the 1990's, ECP was enhanced by the addition of electronically controlled inflation and deflation valves. These valves are connected to three pairs of pneumatic cuffs, which are wrapped around the calves, thighs, and buttocks. The cuffs are sequentially inflated to 300 mm Hg with compressed air from far end to near end as the heart begins to rest in diastole. They are rapidly deflated as the heart begins to beat in systole. A microprocessor determines the moment of diastole and the moment of systole by interpreting the EKG. This microprocessor is what "enhances" regular ECP to make it EECP.

EECP has been validated by clinical trials involving thousands of patients. What have clinical research trials established about the benefits of EECP?

• *EECP almost always increases tolerance for exercise.*[3] If you do EECP, you will feel more like being active.

• *EECP reduces angina in about 85 percent of patients who go through the entire 35 sessions of treatment.*[4] It usually takes at least 15 treatments for angina to get better. Most people notice a change by the thirtieth day they are doing EECP.

• *EECP doesn't increase oxygen supply to tissues throughout the body, but it does seem to reduce oxygen demand by tissues throughout the body.*[5] This means you won't huff and puff as much when you exercise. It also means that your body can tolerate anaerobic exercise better. It will be easier for you, when your doctor approves, to do brief wind sprints as part of your aerobic exercise. I hadn't done sprints in about seven years until I had EECP. Now I do them with every workout.

After EECP, tissues don't need as much oxygen. They get all the oxygen they need. That's when some amazing things happen. The heart's ejection fraction (the percentage of blood inside the heart that it can send out to the rest of the body in one heartbeat) usually goes up. It especially goes up when the damage was on the left side of the heart.[6]

People with blockages of the LAD tolerate exercise better, and their hearts can do more with less oxygen.[7] Diabetics and pre-diabetics develop better blood flow in their arms and legs.[8] They get better control over their blood sugar levels and markers of inflammation.[9] Men being treated for angina recover from erectile dysfunction.[10] When you can move more easily, you aren't as prone to getting depressed. EECP treats depression in men and women who have angina.[11] EECP eases the effects of blockages of the carotid artery.[12] This means that you may see better or overcome brain fog. Before I had a complete set of 35 sessions of EECP, I was having trouble with a condition called amaurosis fugax. My vision would simply come and go because of hardening of my carotid artery. After EECP, this didn't happen. My cardiologist commented that it is possible to grow a collateral vessel for the internal carotid artery in your brain, too. I don't know if that is what happened for me, but I do know I see a lot better than I did before I had EECP.

This is a patient's view of EECP, so I won't try to wade too far into the science. If you are concerned about the science of EECP, you can read the original papers to which I provide citations at the end of this book. But it turns out that EECP doesn't just benefit the heart.

CHAPTER 3:

WHAT ELSE CAN EECP DO FOR YOU?

I have mentioned that when I first started EECP, I was skeptical. The staff at the vascular care center where I got my treatments seemed, well, a little too enthusiastic. Then when I found out what EECP had done for me, I insisted on getting the full 35 treatments.

It turns out that, if anything, the staff at Legacy Heart Care where I was treated were understating the benefits of the procedure. EECP is FDA-approved for cardiovascular care. It's covered by medical insurance. But some patients achieve additional benefits that the heart care center usually does not mention that have been documented in the medical literature.

- *Sports performance.* The Nike Sports Research Lab studied 19 athletes given 35 hours of EECP. They found that the athletes who completed the treatment had better balance, greater O2 consumption, longer time to lactate production ("burn"), and greater exercise tolerance.[1]

- *Cirrhosis of the liver.* EECP improves blood flow to the kidneys in cirrhosis patients waiting for a liver transplant.[2]

- *Diabetes.* EECP reduces insulin resistance during treatment and for three months afterward.[3] This means less insulin is needed to maintain normal blood sugars (and less insulin is available to keep fats locked in fat cells). I personally noticed my blood sugar levels started running about 30 mg/dl lower after my second week of treatment, even though nothing else had changed.

- *Diabetic inflammation.* EECP reduces markers of inflammation in diabetics.[4] This makes red blood cells less "sticky" and less likely to clot. It also slows the ability of cancer cells to form tumors.

- *Diabetic neuropathy.* In interviews of EECP providers for this book, I was told of two cases of patients who had diabetic neuropathy that substantially resolved during treatment. One woman had had no feeling in her feet for 10 years suddenly started feeling ticklish when the medical assistant touched her feet. A man who had diabetic neuropathy for 20 years had a day or two of burning foot pain that was followed by normal sensation's return.

- *Erectile dysfunction.* A study of 35 men who had ED who received EECP found that the average increase in flow through the penile artery was 200 percent, and 11 out of 13 who agreed to measurements had better erectile function.[5]

- *Peripheral vascular disease* (venous insufficiency, varicose veins, and peripheral arterial disease). A study involving 38 volunteers found that a session of EECP increased blood flow similarly to a session of exercise.[6]

- *Restless legs syndrome.* In a small clinical trial without a control group, researchers found that restless legs syndrome essentially disappears for many EECP recipients during treatment, and that the benefits actually improve over the next six months even after EECP treatment is complete.[7]

- *Sudden deafness.* Another German study found that 28 percent of EECP patients who had sudden deafness due to vascular problems improved with EECP, with an average improvement of hearing threshold of 19 dB.

- **Tinnitus**. The same German researchers also found that 47 percent of tinnitus patients receiving EECP had improved symptoms for a full year following treatment.[8]

There are also some benefits that you may experience that aren't documented in the medical literature. Did you lose a lot of weight after you got treated for your heart attack? That is what happens when your heart recovers enough strength to move fluid. You may lose "water weight" when you do EECP.

EECP treatment can also affect your complexion. For me, the extra circulation to my face canceled out some of my age spots. I'm not saying that you should give up your Aveda or Estee Lauder for counterpulsation treatment, but it certainly won't hurt. If you're like me, and you don't use cosmetics (in my generation, it wasn't a guy thing), it may be very noticeable.

And you may notice some changes in the venous insufficiency. Venous insufficiency is a condition that more people have than know about. It's caused by damage to the valves that keep blood flowing through your legs back up to you heart. When these valves don't work, you can have "droopy" legs when you walk. You can have dry, irritated, purple skin on your lower legs. These splotches of purple skin can progress to open wounds that don't heal.

I've never had peripheral arterial disease (PAD), but I have had some major problems with venous insufficiency. When I started EECP, I carried a cane to prop myself up when I left my home, for all the times I would have to stand and wait somewhere. Before EECP, standing in line was physically painful. After EECP it wasn't. One leg was bigger than the other due to swelling. After EECP it wasn't. And I didn't need a cane to get around.

EECP can do some remarkable things. But there are some people who can't have it.

CHAPTER 4:
CAN EVERYBODY HAVE EECP?

EECP is safe. It's non-invasive. It's drug-free. EECP is appropriate for almost anyone with heart disease, even some kinds of heart patients who would never get a referral to other kinds of cardiac rehabilitation.

People who have pacemakers can get EECP. People who have implanted defibrillators can get the treatment, too. Atrial fibrillation (A-fib) under good control, with a heart rate of 50 to 100 beats per minute, is not a bar to EECP treatment, and you can be cleared for treatment even if you are on a blood thinner.

Most valve disorders, such as a mitral valve prolapse, a leaky mitral, pulmonic, or tricuspid valve, or a "tight" value are not a barrier to EECP. The valve problem will not improve, but EECP will still be beneficial.

Similarly, valve problems in the saphenous veins in the legs that cause venous insufficiency are not a problem for EECP treatment. Symptoms of venous insufficiency may improve. There may be less redness or swelling. But that's because EECP is something like "support hose on steroids," not because venous valves have repaired themselves.

Each heart is unique, but enhanced external counterpulsation therapy, EECP, not just an earlier version of the technique called "ECP," automatically takes individual differences into account. Your heart controls the pace of the treatment, rather than the other way around. The pressure cuffs inflate when your heart is at rest. They deflate when your heart presses blood outward into your body. The rhythm of the treatment is determined by the rhythm of your heart.

By creating a counter flow to your circulatory system, EECP provides your aorta with up to 93 percent more oxygen and nutrients. It gives your heart a 28 percent boost in oxygen and nutrients for the length of the session.[1] Whatever your degree of fitness, EECP kicks you up to the next level. But not everyone is ready for EECP.

Recent invasive heart procedures may require waiting time. You can have EECP as soon as about a week after you have a heart catheterization, angioplasty, or stent placement. The only requirement is that incision site into your femoral artery should be healed. If the incision site is red, oozy, or tender to the touch, you should wait until it has been healed. The wrap around the upper thigh goes all the way to the groin, so if an incision site in your groin is not completely healed, the pressure cuff will be very uncomfortable.

There is a longer waiting time after bypass surgery. It's necessary for the incisions where leg veins were harvested to heal completely before you have EECP.

Your surgeon will want to wait until you are in stable condition, not needing to go back to the hospital, making steady progress. It may be two or three months after bypass surgery before you can have EECP.

EECP is safe for most people who have a history with blood clotting problems. It actually makes the blood less likely to clot. Blood clots when it is stagnant. EECP increases circulation so blood is less likely to clot. However, special situations require special attention.

A history of blood clots in the leg requires special attention. If you have a history of deep vein thrombosis (DVT), usually you can have EECP if your doctor confirms that your blood clotting factors are under good control. My doctor ordered an ultrasound of the veins in my leg just to make sure. If you currently have a blood clot, of course, you won't get EECP.

Blood thinners usually are not a problem. EECP pressure cuffs go all the way around your leg, so any downward pressure in one location is balanced by "upward" pressure on the other side of the leg. The net pressure on your leg is no more than a good poke with your finger. EECP does not cause bleeding, but just to make sure there are no problems should a pressure cuff become lose or get taken off while the pressure is still running, most EECP centers look for your INR to be below 3.0 to 3.5.

A Greenfield filter is not a bar to EECP. A Greenfield filter is designed to catch blood clots before they go into the aorta. There's no special problem with having EECP even if you have the device. But there are conditions that are an absolute bar to having enhanced external counterpulsation therapy.

Fever has to go down before you can have EECP.
Running a temperature is a sign that your body is fighting
infection. EECP increases circulation to the heart. You
don't want to drive the microorganism causing the
infection into your heart, so you cannot have EECP until
your fever goes down. If you know you have a fever on a
day you are scheduled for EECP, call your provider to
confirm your status and be ready to reschedule your
session.

**Cellulitis in your lower legs is a strong reason not
to have EECP.** Cellulitis is sometimes a "tunneling"
infection. You don't want to press the capillaries in your
lower leg so that the bacteria causing cellulitis can more
easily move up your leg. If you have pink, tender skin on
your legs with heat and swelling, let your provider know.
They may not always check for every single session. There
is only one patient in the medical literature who developed
cellulitis and toxic shock syndrome after EECP treatment,[2]
and I happen to know another, but both patients did well
with EECP after antibiotic treatment. It was just necessary
to get the infection under control first.

**Abdominal aortic aneurysm, also known as AAA is
a contraindication for EECP**. If you have an abdominal
aortic aneurysm of 5 cm diameter or greater, your doctor
will usually insist on having it repaired before you have any
kind of counterpulsation treatment. If you have already had
AAA repair, then the EECP center may want you to have a
CT scan to make sure that there are not any tiny tears in
your aorta that could leak and cause future problems.
These issues have to be resolved before you have EECP.

**Severe aortic insufficiency is a bar to treatment
with EECP**. This relatively rare condition is diagnosed by
an ultrasound of the heart. Since EECP sends blood back

into the aorta between heartbeats, a weak aorta could be made weaker by treatment. After the aorta has been surgically repaired, then EECP treatment is possible.

Open wounds have to heal before you have EECP, with one notable exception. Any cut, abrasion, burn, or tear of the skin that would be under a pressure cuff has to heal before EECP treatment can begin. However, non-healing diabetic wounds are not a barrier to EECP. They may even heal during treatment as circulation is increased.

Three more conditions also prevent EECP treatment:

Hemophilia. People with this rare blood clotting disorder cannot receive EECP.

Uncontrolled high blood pressure. Most doctors won't approve EECP if blood pressure exceeds 180/100. Your blood pressure will be checked before and after each session.

Pregnancy. Doctors don't really know what effects of increasing blood flow through the placenta have on the unborn. To be safe, EECP is not offered to women who are pregnant.

CHAPTER 5:

HOW TO BE SURE YOU SUCCEED WITH EECP

Heart disease is a whole-body illness. EECP is a whole-body treatment. EECP is like a highly concentrated workout in a heart health gym, only the cuffs are doing all the work for you while you are lying down, watching TV, listening to music, or taking a nap.

EECP doesn't give you all the benefits of a regular workout. It won't burn very many calories. It won't change your metabolic rate. But it will give you all the cardiovascular benefits of a week at the gym in a single one-hour session that you do 35 times in over seven weeks. It keeps your heart bathed in oxygen and nutrients. It stimulates your blood vessels to grow. And it has a beneficial effect on just about every aspect of your health that is affected by your heart's health. So what do you need to do to get the most from EECP?

Repetition is the key. Everybody knows that one trip to the gym isn't going to give you a sleek physique and powerful muscles. If you do a hard workout just once and then veg out on the couch for six months, you may get some temporarily sore muscles, but you will not have done anything to give yourself new pep and energy. Exercise requires repetition to work. You have to work at active exercise to enjoy its benefits for your body.

You don't have to work at EECP. EECP is passive exercise. It does the work for you. You do have to show up, however, and stick your treatment schedule for your body to get the message that it needs to change.

EECP consists of 35 one-hour sessions. That number was not selected randomly. When Chinese doctors started studying EECP, they gave their patients stress tests after every 12 treatments. They found that coronary function improved after 12, 24, and 36 sessions, but the benefits of EECP maxed out after six weeks of six treatments per day.[1] Chinese clinics are typically open six days a week, but American and European clinics typically are closed on the weekend, so they offer 35 treatments over seven weeks rather than 36 treatments over six. All of the research studies conducted on "EECP" using equipment manufactured by Vasotech have been done with 35 treatments, so every program in the US and Europe is 35 treatments long.

You can double up. Not every EECP program is seven weeks long, however. After you have had your first two weeks of treatment, your treatment center may be able to accommodate you for two treatments a day, as long as you have an hour to rest between sessions. *However, doubling up one day does not mean you can skip the next day.* Constant stimulation of the angiogenic growth factors and constant reduction of the endothelin inflammation factors discussed in Chapter 2 is essential to rerouting blood flow and growing new blood vessels. Most programs will allow for seven absences over seven weeks, rescheduling your treatments when emergencies or illness force you to miss, but if you make a habit of missing your sessions, you are likely to be dropped from treatment.

Improvements are usually obvious after 15 to 20 treatments. Sometimes patients start feeling markedly better after one week of EECP. I grew a new coronary artery after just 10 treatments, a later catheterization proved. Most people start feeling changes after 15 to 20 treatments.

What kinds of changes will you probably feel after you have EECP? You probably will be able to walk farther and walk faster. If you use nitroglycerin on a regular basis, you will probably use less. You may lose a little water weight as your circulation improves. You might be able to mow the lawn or pick up the couch or make love. As so many programs advise, your results will vary.

Taking more than 35 treatments is possible. When medical researchers do clinical trials, they choose participants who meet a narrow range of qualifications that limit the number of variables in the study. In the real world, there are about as many different health concerns as there are people who need EECP. Some people simply need more than 35 treatments to get maximum benefits:

Most people don't have a problem with the pressure cuffs used in EECP, but some people do. They may need a few days up to two weeks to gradually get used to the full pressure needed to reverse enough blood flow to cause the hormonal changes that repair arteries and reroute circulation. Maybe they will need full-pressure treatments for less than the full hour. Maybe they will need low-pressure treatments for the usual hour session. Either way, they need to get the full pressure of the cuffs (260 mm of mercury) for the full hour to get the vascular benefits for which the treatment is designed. They may need more than 35 treatments.

People who have peripheral arterial disease PAD are slower to respond to EECP. They simply don't have as much blood flowing to their legs to be pumped back toward the heart. The first two or three weeks are needed to improve circulation in the legs, and then EECP can improve circulation to the heart.

Some people with advanced heart disease don't respond to just 35 treatments. A study done in the late 1990's found that 86 percent of patients who had a bypass on just one artery had improved circulation after the standard course of EECP. When the doctors analyzed the results for patients who had had two bypasses, they found that 85 percent had better circulation after 35 treatments. When the doctors looked at the data for patients who had had three bypasses, only 53 percent were better after 35 treatments.[2] However, the answer isn't that these patients shouldn't do EECP at all. It's that they should try more than 35 sessions.

I personally needed 45 sessions to really start feeling good. But I have eight stents, including a stent inside a stent inside a stent inside a stent in the same segment of the same artery. I am hoping I have maxed out on stents with the help of EECP.

Certain health conditions require special attention. Just as people come to EECP with different degrees of cardiovascular damage, they deal with different non-vascular diseases. Certain diseases require a different approach for success with EECP.

People over 80. EECP tends to get good results in the elderly. Dr. Debra Braverman followed 24 of her patients who had an average age of just under 85 years. A year after treatment, 23 continued to have improved quality of life and increased activity level. None experienced adverse symptoms related to EECP.[3] The International EECP Patient Registry tracked results of treatment for 249 patients over 80 years of age. In this group, 76 percent reported improved activity levels at the conclusion of their treatment, and 81 reported that their improved activity levels continued one year later.[4] Octogenarians are more prone to falls, problems with blood clotting factors, and infections, and these also have to be monitored even after they have EECP. In particular, increased activity can be a problem in the elderly who suffer dementia. Their caregivers may have to take a new ability to wander away or get into situations where falls are possible into account.

Women. On the whole women respond to EECP as well or better than men. However, women do not respond to percutaneous coronary intervention (angioplasty and stenting) the same way as men. Women tend to have smaller coronary arteries, and more complications after procedures in the cath lab.[5] The also suffer more complications after bypass surgery. Women are more likely than men to have to go back into the hospital after bypass surgery. They are more likely to suffer setbacks in the functional abilities. They are more likely to develop depression.[6] Women may be well enough for EECP and benefit from it, but just getting EECP is not a reason to reduce active monitoring for complications, especially not in women.

People who are exposed to second-hand smoke. EECP patients who live with smokers are less likely to experience benefits early in treatment. This makes them less inclined to complete treatment. They also get less relief from angina. If you live with someone who smokes, expect to see results later rather than sooner. A strong majority (69 percent, in one study) of people who live with smokers experience significant improvement in angina, one "class" or more. But a little less than a third of people who live with smokers don't get a full reduction of angina in just 35 treatments. They still improve, but not as dramatically.[7]

People who suffer depression. Heart disease is depressing. It's especially depressing in people who develop it early in life, in their forties or even sooner. A study in Denmark focusing on 50 patients who had heart disease found that EECP is a good treatment for depression, and the improvement in depression occurs even before the improvement in chest pain.[8] If you have depression, it's best to plan for success. Talk with your doctor about the best way to manage antidepressants if you start feeling naturally better with EECP.

People who suffer "brain fog" with congestive heart failure. Turkish researchers studied the effects of EECP on cognitive function in people over 60 who had both congestive heart failure and cognitive issues. They found that EECP improved most practical brain functions except vision and verbal expression. The ability to remember, to find one's way around, to control emotions and to make good decisions was improved by EECP.[9] Surely that's a good thing, right? At the end of treatment it certainly is. It's during treatment, when there has been just a little improvement yet, that additional caution may be needed.

People who have diabetes. I have had insulin-dependent diabetes since I caught a viral infection when I was 40. After about six weeks of EECP, I noticed my blood sugar levels at night were getting down into the 60's (60 mg/dl, or around 3.5 mmol/L). That's not low enough to cause serious problems, but it is low enough to require a change in routine. One study found that diabetic patients developed better circulation to their muscles, so their bodies used more glucose, and blood sugar levels were on average 28 mg/dl (about 1.5 mmol/L) lower.[10] It's always best to test rather than guess how your blood sugar levels are doing, and if you are a diabetic on EECP, you definitely need to take blood sugar reading before bed.

People who have Prinzmetal's variant angina. If you have never heard of Prinzmetal's variant angina, chances are you don't have it. Typical angina is aggravated by activity. Prinzmetal's occurs at rest. Cardiologists usually don't have experience in treating it with EECP. However, one patient who had the disease and got EECP had 81 hospitalizations in two years before EECP, and just two hospitalizations in the two years after EECP.[11]

There are also some considerations that just about every EECP patient has to consider.

Repeating EECP treatment. Heart treatments, even bypass, angioplasty, and stents, are seldom one-and-done. That's because heart disease is usually chronic and progressive. It's not unusual for heart patients to have to make complex decisions about risky and expensive procedures more than once. I myself had seven stent procedures that placed eight stents before I finally decided I just wasn't going to have another. For me, the issue was still quality of life, but stents just weren't working. I needed something else. Similar decisions drive many people to EECP.

EECP after angioplasty or stent procedures. Dr. Debra Braverman reports that 30 percent of her patients experienced restenosis (closing) of arteries in the first six months after angioplasty or stent placement. I had a stent fail after just six weeks. Its replacement failed after about six days.

Because angioplasty and stents often fail to produce lasting results, they are often repeated. The problem is that a second, third, fourth, or fifth procedure does not necessarily help very long. Stent procedures can cause the buildup of scar tissue. Angioplasty may not completely remove the plaque blocking an artery. Both procedures can change the "plumbing" of the coronary arteries so that your original blood vessels interact with your collateral blood vessels in unexpected ways. Opening one the arteries you were born with may drain a collateral artery so that it closes. Repeated angioplasty or stents may simply move the area of oxygen deprivation from one part of your heart to another.

The changes in your blood vessels from EECP are much faster than those that you could get from working out in the gym, but they are much slower than the changes you get from angioplasty or stenting. In EECP, your body develops the new blood vessels it needs and only the new blood vessels it needs. If your arteries are open enough that blood does not flow backward during your treatment, then those blood vessels don't release the growth factors that produce new arteries.

The International EECP Patient Registry contains data on patients who had angioplasty or a stent that failed compared to patients who tried EECP first. It's a lot more common just to go ahead and get angioplasty and/or a stent that it is to wait to see how 35 sessions of EECP work out. However, the registry had data on 315 patients who were candidates for interventional procedures but opted to get EECP before going to the cath lab. Researchers compared their experiences with those of 3,179 patients who tried angioplasty and/or stents first that failed.

The data in the registry showed that both groups benefited from EECP. Both groups had about the same reduction in angina. Both groups decreased their use of nitroglycerin at about the same rates. Both groups continued to improve for six months even after they completed EECP. However, 315 patients never had to have angioplasty or stents because EECP was enough of them.[12]

EECP after bypass surgery. Grafted blood vessels tend to close over time. The doctor who did a catheterization on my dad 10 years after he had a triple bypass commented that he had been left with "just a thread" of an LAD. My dad did not have an opportunity to get EECP. But if he had, chances are it still would have helped even after his three bypass grafts had closed up again.

Doctors at the State University of New York at Stony Brook compared the outcome of 35 patients who had been offered bypass surgery but chose to get EECP first with the outcome of 25 patients who had bypass grafts that failed and then decided to get EECP. All 60 patients had blockages greater than 70 percent. The study found that patients who had one or two blockages who didn't get bypass surgery did just as well as patients who had one or two failed bypass grafts, both groups after EECP. Not absolutely every patient in either group benefited from EECP, but 88 percent of those who had *not* had bypass surgery did. This compared to 80 percent success among those who had already had bypass surgery.

The researchers were even more surprised that patients who had three blockages but had bypass surgery that failed actually fared a lot better than patients who had not had bypass surgery yet. Among those who had already had three failed bypass grafts, 80 percent improved with EECP.[13] Of course, if you have had a bypass operation and you feel fine, you probably aren't going to seek EECP. But maybe you should.

What about EECP after EECP? At the University of California Medical Center at San Francisco, a little under 20 percent of EECP patients come back for another round of treatments in two years or less. Other studies have found that about 40 percent of EECP patients will come back in five years or less.

Heart disease is systemic, chronic, and progressive. It can snatch away the gains you make in one year so that you need more treatment the next. That's why it is extremely important to work with your cardiologist to achieve ongoing heart health. Diet and exercise make a difference.

CHAPTER 6. DIET AND EECP

Diet has never been a major concern in EECP treatment. The improvements for enhanced external counterpulsation therapy do not depend on how well you stick to your prescribed diet plan. If they did, probably a lot fewer people would benefit from the program.

Fortunately for most of us, EECP improves the state of health you have now. But that doesn't mean that a few changes in diet can't help you do better. In this chapter I'll suggest some simple additions to your diet a major subtraction, and a general consideration. There is nothing complicated about this "EECP Diet."

Make three simple additions to your heart-healthy diet. If you are old enough to remember the Popeye cartoons, you undoubtedly recall his famous byline: "I'm strong to the finich (finish) 'cause I eat my spinach, I'm Popeye the sailor man!"

Popeye could have added, "I don't eat me sweets but I do eat me beets." Spinach and beets are in the same plant family. These two foods share some biochemical and nutritional characteristics. Let's start with beets.

My late mama served pickled beets at nearly every meal except breakfast. I wouldn't have been surprised if she had put them on ice cream (although except when she was pregnant with my younger brother, I never saw her do this). It turns out that there is scientific confirmation of how beets help heart health.

A study conducted by scientists in Australia, Iran, and the Southern University Agricultural Research and Extension Center in Baton Rouge, Louisiana asked volunteers to consume either 250 ml (about a cup) of beet juice or 250 grams (a little over half a pound) of cooked beets every day for two weeks. At the end of the two weeks, the volunteers switched from beet juice to beet root or vice versa. Both cooked beets and beet juice improved blood flow, although beet juice was slightly more effective than cooked beet root. Beet juice but not cooked beats also lowered both total cholesterol and LDL. However, volunteers also had lower HDL when they consumed beet juice.[1]

A study of well-conditioned soccer players confirmed that the contribution of beet juice to improved vascular flow is in its nitrate content.[2] This would make drinking beet juice a little like taking Imdur or Imzo or nitroglycerin pills, only without the headaches.

Another study of young male athletes found that adding nitrates to the diet, in an amount similar to the nitrates you would get from eating 5 servings of vegetables a day, helped muscles do more work with less oxygen.[3] Beets and related plants like spinach are the best easy-to-get vegetables for dietary nitrates.

So what's not to love about beets? The detail from the research studies that promoters of beet powder supplements tend to overlook is that the more in-shape you are, the more you respond to dietary nitrate. Beets do a body good, but they do more good when the body is already in good physical fit. All this means for people who choose EECP is that the longer you add beets to your diet, the better you will feel.

Of course, not everyone likes beets. If you don't eat beets, maybe you will eat spinach. Scientists at the Karolinska Institute in Stockholm have found that the nitrates in spinach help cells function better under conditions of oxygen deprivation. Feeding volunteer athletes 200 to 300 grams of spinach a day (that's about 1/2 to 2/3 pound, and it's a lot) decreased oxygen needs during exercise.[4]

This is particularly valuable to people who have diabetes. When your muscle operates under low-oxygen conditions, it burns up to 35 times more glucose than normal. This helps give lower-intensity exercise the same ability to lower your blood sugar levels as wind sprints and power lifting. Unless you start eating those bulk boxes of spinach you sometimes see in the produce section you aren't likely to become hypoglycemic or to develop unusually low blood pressure, but adding spinach to your daily diet can be as helpful as many of the medications you take.

If you just don't "do" beets or spinach, lettuce is the next best thing. Lettuce provides smaller amounts of the nitrates that help improve coronary circulation. Almost any leafy green is good for your heart, as is the lowly potato. However, make it a habit to eat your spuds boiled, not fried or baked with the butter and cheese. There's a very specific reason for that.

Avoid high-fat meals, but not because they are high in cholesterol. Cholesterol has long been the bugaboo of cardiovascular care. There are longstanding misconceptions about the role of cholesterol in atherosclerosis. There are widespread misunderstandings about what LDL and HDL numbers mean and whether you can trust your lab results. The reason you probably really do need to be taking a statin is for fighting inflammation, not for lowering your cholesterol. But you still need to avoid high-fat meals. Here's why.

A high-fat, high-calorie meal reduces the ability of your arteries to "go with the flow." For up to eight hours after you eat a high-fat meal, your arteries cannot as easily relax to accommodate increase blood flow. This means that if you have to do physical work, you go the gym, or you just get very excited, your blood pressure will spike because your arteries have less "flow mediated dilation." They can't "go with the flow" as long as tiny particles of fat and high concentrations of triglyceride from excess carbohydrate are floating through your blood stream.[5]

When researchers have studied the effects of high-fat, high-energy meals, they usually have given volunteers some kind of "shake" made with cream, eggs, and lots of sugar. You can translate this into your eating habits. Don't have the crème brûlée after you chomp down a ribeye. Skip the fries with your burger. Or skip the burger altogether. Small amounts of fat aren't deadly if they come with low-calorie meals. High-calorie meals may play havoc with your blood sugar levels but they won't create a sludge flowing through your arteries unless they contain lots of fat. But as a general rule, it's always best to save something for next time. Don't eat all your favorite foods all at once. You will save your heart a potentially toxic overload.

Don't go nuts over fruit and nuts, but consider adding them to your diet. You have probably heard of the heart-healthy Mediterranean diet. It's the diet that emphasizes olive oil, fresh vegetables, and fish, with minimal amounts of bread, almost no sweets except an occasional spoonful of honey, and certainly no fast foods. I won't repeat what you probably have already heard (and if you want more information, please visit my website myeecp.com), but I will add an important additional finding from recent research:

Fortifying a Mediterranean diet with either extra virgin olive oil or healthy nuts (almonds, walnuts, and hazelnuts have been tested in clinical trials) resulted in far lower levels of the markers of inflammation (IL-1β, IL-5, IL-7, IL-12p70, IL-18, TNF-α, IFN-γ, GCSF, GMCSF, and ENA78) that can transform a stable cholesterol plaque into a dangerous, potentially ruptured cholesterol plaque.[6]

In a five-year study involving 7447 people in Spain, the research team either sent each participant's family a liter of high-quality Spanish extra-virgin olive oil every week, or 200 grams (about 8 oz) of nuts, or both. They found that either olive oil or nuts had a beneficial effect on atherosclerosis. The research team did not tell the participants what else to eat or how to exercise or ask them to count calories. They just gave the participants healthy foods and let them decide on their own how to eat them. They did not worry about weight, although a number of studies have found that when people eat more nuts, they don't gain more weight, because they are more satisfied and not as hungry. Of course, if you are allergic to nuts, don't eat them.

What about fruit? It's true that fruit is a source of fructose. You have probably heard that fructose is horrible for your health. That's because corn syrup is more than 50 percent fructose, and American soft drinks and snack desserts practically float in high-fructose corn syrup. If you get 300, 400, 500, or even more calories from high-fructose corn syrup every day, you will overwhelm your body's ability to store excess sugar as fat.

However, even though fruit contains fructose, it's not a very abundant source of fructose. There's a lot less sugar in an apple than there is in a regular Coke. A Big Gulp at your neighborhood 7-11 might have as much as 10 times as much fructose as a piece of fruit.

Small amounts of fructose aren't harmful. They can "prime" the liver to deal with the glucose released from other foods. Small amounts of fructose even seem to protect blood vessels from the surge of endothelin that comes after a fatty meal. By "small," I mean about two servings of fruit a day, or about 100 calories a day from fruit. And no high-fructose corn syrup.

From time to time researchers study the potential of adding a piece of fruit to a high-fat, high-calorie meal to see if the fructose in the fruit somehow offsets the bad effects of the fat and calories on the cardiovascular system. Time and time again studies produce results that are "almost" significant. It seems that fruit could be generally helpful, but the science just isn't there. Nonetheless, a piece of fruit now and then, unless you are on a ketogenic diet, may help your body deal with the occasional excesses of high fat and high calories. Just have fruit instead of dessert.

CHAPTER 7:
WHAT DO YOU DO AFTER EECP?

Exercise does amazing things. In fact, you could use accomplish the same things with exercise that you do with EECP, only a lot more slowly.

Now that I have had EECP, I am maintaining my gains with a similar program. I just don't do all of my exercise on a stationary bike. As I mentioned earlier in this book, I have decided "no more knife guys." I feel good. I think I'm on the path that will keep me healthy and surgery-free now.

So what's the catch? Two hours of exercise every day does you the same good as EECP, but if you have already had a heart attack or you are recovering from angioplasty, stenting, or bypass, you need something like EECP to be able to do the two hours of exercise.

Exercise is especially good for you after you have EECP. After you have EECP, you will have more energy for exercise. You will enjoy exercise more. You will be less likely to suffer the chest pain of angina—and I will have a few words about how to avoid it later in this chapter—and you will have a better quality of life. But to sustain that new quality of life you have to get moving.

You just don't have to move really fast.

When you are having a heart attack right now, it really is a good idea to have cardiovascular intervention. Multiple clinical studies show that percutaneous coronary intervention extends life and prevents future complications in emergency situations.[1]

Once you symptoms are stable, exercise is better than getting another stent. Clinical studies have shown that a combination of "optimal medical therapy," getting all the right medications, plus exercise is a superior treatment for blockages of the coronary arteries than stenting (percutaneous coronary intervention).

The right medication plus exercise results in fewer future heart attacks than angioplasty or stents. The right medication plus exercise results in fewer future strokes than angioplasty or stents. The right medication plus exercise results in fewer deaths over a period of five years than angioplasty or stents. If you get the medication you need plus the exercise you need, you are less likely to go to the hospital. You are more likely to enjoy sustained quality of life.[2]

Exercise is essential, but it doesn't have to be hard. So how hard do you have to work out to develop new collateral arteries with exercise? And how long?

The EXCITE trial in Germany assigned 20 patients with atherosclerosis to do *high-intensity exercise* two hours a day, five days a week, for four weeks. It assigned another 20 patients with atherosclerosis to do *moderate-intensity exercise* two hours a day, five days a week, for four weeks. And it told a control group of another 20 patients not to do any exercise at all. All of the exercise was done on a stationary bike, so the results would not be swayed by choice of exercise.

How intense were "high-intensity" and "moderate-intensity" exercise?

"High-intensity" exercise was defined as working out hard enough to have a pulse rate 90 percent of what would cause chest pain (angina). "Moderate-intensity" exercise was 60 percent of this maximum pulse rate. If you have heart issues, it turns out that 60 percent of the heart beats per minute that would trigger an attack of angina usually is a comfortable pace, maybe 85 to 100 beats per minute. It's not "hard" exercise at all. The German study required participants to exercise for 30 minutes four times a day, two hours a day in all, five days a week, under close supervision.

So who got better faster? It turned out that moderate exercise was just as effective as high-intensity exercise. You don't have to work out hard to get new collaterals. You do have to work out a lot, or at least most of us consider two hours a day in four sessions to be a lot.

The study involved continuous exercise. This is exercise you do without stopping. And it involved eccentric exercise. "Eccentric exercise" does not mean something like extreme ironing or naked skydiving. "Eccentric" just means that the exercise involves pushing a limb away from the body and bringing it back. When you pedal a stationary bicycle (or a regular bicycle), or your use an elliptical machine, or you snow ski or do pole walking or you swim, you push legs and/or arms away from your body and you bring them back. This creates a counter flow to you usual circulation. It triggers the same kinds of changes as EECP.

Do this for just four weeks, and your circulatory system will get the message that it needs to build new blood vessels.[3]

You just don't have to spend as much time, or energy, when you do EECP. However, it helps to do a passive exercise like EECP first while you are recovering from cardiovascular procedures. What's passive exercise again?

It's really easy exercise. You get exercise, but a machine or another person is doing the work for you. EECP is the best passive exercise for cardiovascular health, but it's not the only one. Here are some examples.

It's only a slight exaggeration to say that **whole body vibration training** shakes you back into shape. It reduces arterial stiffness and increases muscle strength,[4] although it doesn't put any strain on the heart. It won't make your heart beat faster or raise your blood pressure.[5] Even if you don't have enough breathing capacity to do active exercise, for example, you suffer chronic. Some gyms have vibration equipment, but home models are available for $150 to $3500.

Whole body vibration is particularly helpful for increasing knee and thigh strength.[6] It tends to increase muscle mass (usually by 2 to 4 percent) and reduce fat mass (also usually by 2 to 4 percent) without active exercise or dieting.[7] And like EECP, it reduces the production of endothelin, the hormone that makes the linings of blood vessels tighten and causes blood pressure to go up.[8] Also like EECP, it triggers increased production of nitric oxide (NO), which enables blood vessels to relax. [9]

Passive resistance exercise takes your arms and legs through an appropriate range of motion. It can be done for you by a therapist, or with a special machine set for your needs and limitations. This form of exercise is something you can do even if you are confined to bed or a wheelchair.

The **Huber Motion Lab** can be very helpful in strengthening the muscles you use when you are standing. Your response to Huber Motion Training depends on your cardiovascular fitness, but these workouts will not change your arterial stiffness, blood pressure, or ejection fraction, and they won't help you develop new collaterals.

The most familiar form of passive exercise you receive from another person is **massage**. There is scientific evidence that Swedish massage lowers blood pressure. A study involving women with high blood pressure found that four one-hour Swedish massage sessions over four weeks lowered systolic pressure (the first number) on average 12 points (mm Hg), and lowered diastolic blood pressure (the second number) on average five points. Swedish massage also lowers the production of endothelin, about twice as much as taking a nap.[10] The benefits of Swedish massage only last about 72 hours, however, so it's optimal to have two massages a week.[11]

This isn't to say that other styles of massage are not equally helpful. It just happens that cardiovascular researchers studied Swedish massage.

Active exercise does not have to strenuous, either.

There is probably no simpler exercise than *prāṇāyāma*, the **breathing exercise from yoga**. The important thing to remember about any kind of breathing exercise is that slow breathing exercises help the heart, while fast breathing exercises produce other kinds of benefits. With apologies to those who have spent many years mastering yoga and who are vastly more knowledgeable than I, I'll offer a crass over-simplification of how it's done;

- Take an easy short breath in through your nose.
- Take an easy long breath out through your mouth.

Of course, there are left-nostril, right-nostril, alternate-nostril and other techniques of prāṇāyāma, but the effect of them can be summed up in a simple statement: Slow breathing exercises slow down the pulse and lower blood pressure to healthy levels. Fast breathing exercises are for lung capacity.[12]

Bhrāmarī prāṇāyāma is a breathing exercise involves breathing in through both nostrils and making a buzzing sound (like a bee) when exhaling. Most people can overcome the effects of emotional stress on blood pressure and pulse rate by doing the exercise for five minutes.[13]

Praṇava prāṇāyāma is a deep breathing exercise that, like EECP, increases production of nitric oxide.[14] This action opens arteries and lowers blood pressure. Doing yogic exercises is like taking nitroglycerin or nitrates, but never causes side effects or dangerous drug interactions.

Other yogic breathing techniques have similar benefits. Just about anyone can do them. They require no special equipment. You can do them anytime, anywhere. It's best to get some instruction from an expert when you are beginning, but there are YouTube videos, DVDs, and classes.

Only slightly more strenuous are **grip strength exercises**. Not everyone can do them, but most people can. The exercises you do to build grip strength will not build new collateral arteries, but they send blood, oxygen, and nutrients through existing collateral arteries. It only takes three minutes of this kind of exercise to make a difference in your collateral circulation.[15]

Then there is a range of exercises that are more fun, but take longer, generally months instead of weeks, to produce cardiovascular benefits. Here is a list of exercises in order of how long it takes to see results:

- **Walking** won't create new collateral blood vessels, but it will generally make it possible for your whole body to increase blood flow with less effort. Walking also usually raises HDL and lowers LDL and triglycerides. You need to walk for 30 minutes a day, five days a week, for six weeks to see benefits.[16]

- **Swimming** lowers blood pressure. You need to swim for 30 minutes three times a week for 10 weeks to see a change.[17]

- **Low-impact aerobics**, such as dancercise, usually increases blood flow in noticeable ways after three months of three sessions a week, 60 minutes each.[18]

- **Tai chi** helps you with "water weight." It improves balance. Cardiovascular benefits such as lower blood pressure usually take three months of three sessions a week, 60 minutes each.[19]

- **Yoga** requires daily practice to produce lasting benefits (that would continue even if you stopped). Typically you would need to do 60 minutes a day every day for three months.[20]

- **Strength training** may have you feeling better and looking good in just a few weeks, but lower blood pressure and a slower, more athletic heart rate usually come after four months of three sessions a week, 60 minutes each.[21]

EECP is the most efficient form of exercise for cardiovascular rehabilitation. In terms of hours you need to spend doing it, it's the fastest form of exercise for cardiovascular rehabilitation. But after you have finished your 35 sessions of EECP, just keep doing some kind of exercise. You will feel better. You will look better. Your whole life will go more smoothly as you preserve your gains from EECP.

FREQUENTLY ASKED QUESTIONS

I have assembled a collection of questions and answers that come up frequently in EECP. I'm not a doctor so these answers are not medical advice, but they do reflect medical advice given by doctors to EECP patients or my personal experience (which I identify as such). Your doctor is always your first, last, and best source of guidance for your health decisions. However, you may find some important questions you had not considered here.

What does the acronym EECP stand for?

Enhanced external counterpulsation therapy. This is actually a trademarked term. It always refers to the use of "enhanced" technology provided by Vasotech. This enhanced method of ECP incorporates microprocessors and controllers to time the inflation and deflation of the pressure cuffs.

So that means there's also such a thing as ECP?

Yes, if you were getting the same kind of treatment at one of the thousands of clinics that offer it in India, China, or Turkey, you would probably be getting "ECP."

What does EECP feel like? Does it hurt?

Most people compare EECP to getting a deep tissue massage to your legs. It's not painful for most people. You won't feel anything in your heart or chest. The pressure exerted by the cuffs is not even as much as getting poked by somebody's finger. However, the pressure is applied over a large part of your lower body.

Is there any kind of warm up for EECP?

EECP places equal pressure on your legs from all sides at the same time. That's why you won't injure any muscles with EECP. You don't have to do any kind of warmup before your treatments. However, if you have trouble lying still for an hour, it can help to do the same stretches you might do before you settle into a passenger seat on an airplane or before you do some work at your computer. I did chair yoga for a couple of minutes in the changing room before most of my sessions.

Is it OK to eat or drink before an EECP session?

Legacy Heart Care in Austin is just down the street from a kolache (Czech pastry) shop. I grew up eating kolaches, and I had a weakness for scarfing down a kolache or two on my way to EECP. I didn't have any problems those days I had a little snack before I did my EECP treatment. I did have a problem if I drank a big, fizzy soft drink right before EECP. There was one day the other patients could have heard my digestive tract making a noise like an out of tune trombone for about 10 minutes during my treatment. I suggest avoiding carbonated beverages before EECP.

Is it OK to have caffeine (coffee, tea, sodas) before EECP?

If you usually have a rapid pulse, it is best not to make it even more rapid with a jolt of caffeine in the hour to 90 minutes before your treatment. There were several days that I had a cup of coffee at the kolache shop mentioned above, and the pumping of the EECP cuffs was notably faster because my pulse was notably faster.

Does EECP make your heart beat faster or slower?

No. Your heart determines the pace of treatment, not the other way around. That's what the EKG sensors on your chest are for. They pace the inflation and deflation of the cuffs to send blood back to your heart *between* beats.

What do I wear during EECP?

You will need to exchange your pants or skirt for the tights that the treatment center will provide you. They are not hard to put on, although they are a little tighter than long underwear (and you can use them for winter wear when you have finished EECP). You wear the same shirt or blouse you would ordinarily wear for a casual setting.

What do I wear on my feet during EECP?

Most people wear socks. The EECP cuffs do not cover your feet. Some people go barefoot. If you wear support hose to prevent friction of the cuffs against your skin, you won't wear socks.

What if I'm one of the people who finds EECP just a little too much pressure for comfort?

The main thing is to let your EECP provider know if you are uncomfortable. You will probably be offered bubble wrap, support hose (even if you are a man), or fleece. I've tried two of the three. Bubble wrap left bubble type markings on my skin and it didn't work too well for relieving pressure, either, at least for me. I passed on support hose. Call me old fashioned, but I just couldn't see myself parading out to the EECP room with support hose on my toes. Fleece, however, worked just fine. I was a little uncomfortable without it, but I felt perfectly comfortable once the medical technician put it over a sensitive area.

Can I wear compression stockings (like those you wear for varicose veins or venous insufficiency) while I get EECP?

No, the EECP cuffs are calibrated to deliver a precise amount of pressure at precise locations on your legs to send blood up to your heart between beats. They can't be calibrated for compression stockings, so you have to take them off during treatment.

What do I do while I am getting EECP treatment?

The treatment center will usually provide a large-screen TV with various video and music channels, or you can listen to music or radio through headphones, or you can just take a nap. I got hooked on a Netflix series called Longmire, but otherwise I might have taken a nap.

What if I have to use the restroom during treatment?

You will probably have a bell you can use to get the attention of a technician. Get their attention. They will stop the machinery, unhook your cuffs, and let you go to the restroom. When you come back, they hook you up again restart the pressure cuffs so you can get your full hour of EECP. It's best to avoid this, of course.

What if I have to miss a treatment?

Most treatment centers will make allowances for one absence a week. You still have to have the session, but they will reschedule. If you miss several days in a row without a very good reason, however, they will probably drop you from the program. As I pointed out in Chapter 5, repetition is critical to healing your heart with EECP.

Is EECP really safe? Can it cause a heart attack?

I'll answer the second question first. Not only can EECP not cause a heart attack, it is used as an FDA-approved treatment for a heart attack. The medical literature contains absolutely no reports of deaths caused by EECP.

Has the FDA approved EECP?

The Food and Drug Administration approved EECP for treatment of angina and coronary artery disease and for acute care of a heart attack in 1995. (My father got external counterpulsation therapy during a heart attack in 1995. He was the first patient at his hospital to get it on an emergency basis.) The FDA also approved EECP for the treatment of congestive heart failure in 2002.

How can I pay for EECP?

Medicare, most states' Medicaid, and all health insurance plans in the United States cover EECP. In other countries, it is covered by the national health insurance plan. Insurance companies prefer you get EECP over other kinds of coronary intervention. A full course of EECP, with the doctor's fees for supervision, costs your insurance company $3000 to $5000. That's a lot less than the $25,000 to $100,000 or even more for angioplasty and stents.

Do insurance companies make it a hassle to get EECP approved?

You betcha'. But insurance companies put up hurdles for all kinds of treatment. Your EECP provider will have secured pre-approval before your treatment, and it is unlikely they will interrupt your treatment should questions arise after your treatment has started. *However, if you fail to report for too many of your scheduled treatments, you may lose your insurance approval.*

Are there any age limits for EECP?

In my very limited experience (I've only met maybe 100 people who have had EECP in person), I have met patients as young as 44 and as mature as 87. Dr. Debra Braverman reported she had patients ranging in age from 36 to 97. Many EECP patients are over 80.

Does absolutely everyone feel better after EECP?

No, about 80 percent of people who get EECP report better quality of life after 35 sessions of EECP. Some people are worn out by fitting EECP into their schedule and may feel better if they just stick to the 35 sessions. And there are some people for whom EECP isn't particularly helpful. There are some indications (see the comment on congestive heart failure below) that genetics play a role in how you react to EECP. Most people respond. A minority do not.

Will EECP help me lose weight?

As your heart gets stronger, your body may shed a few pounds of water weight. You don't burn a lot of calories during EECP. After all, it is *passive* exercise. However, you may feel like more activity, and that may help you lose weight if you don't also eat more.

Is EECP helpful for congestive heart failure?

A study at the prestigious Karolinska Institute in Sweden published in 2016 reported that EECP stimulates genes that create new heart muscle. The study said the effect was small but measurable.

I have congestive heart failure. I have not had a heart attack. Is EECP appropriate for me?

Your doctor is your best source of advice, but EECP is used to treat congestive heart failure of any cause.

Will EECP have any effect on my cholesterol levels?

EECP will not raise or lower your cholesterol levels. However, there 10 studies that suggest that EECP will stop inflammatory processes from transforming cholesterol into atherosclerotic plaques in the linings of your arteries, and prevent your arteries from growing tissue over the plaques you already have that make your arteries narrower.

Will EECP have any effect on my blood sugar levels?

My blood sugar levels were markedly lower, 30 mg/dl both before and after meals, after EECP treatment. This wasn't enough to cause hypoglycemia, but I did have to change my diabetes routine *because I was getting more exercise* (and not just walking up to the kolache shop). I can't tell you how EECP will affect *your* blood sugar levels, but I suggest that you make sure you test your blood sugars as often as your doctor tells you need to. You may be pleasantly surprised.

Does EECP have any effect on hormone levels?

A Turkish study found that **thyroid stimulating hormone** (TSH) tended to increase about 1 mIU/L during EECP therapy. This could make a difference in *hyper*thyroidism (too much thyroid activity) but is less likely to make a difference in *hypo*thyroidism (not enough thyroid activity). Ask your primary care provider to follow your

TSH before and after treatment, but don't expect huge change.

Can I skip medications if I do EECP?

Absolutely not. You need to continue all your prescribed medications while you do EECP. It is particularly important that you remember to take your beta-blocker, since you can't have EECP if your pulse goes over 100 beats per minute.

Could counterpulsation therapy be done with massage, manual massage, by people, not by machines?

This would not be "enhanced" external counterpulsation therapy, but it is possible to approximate the effects of counterpulsation therapy by people with appropriate training. My father got counterpulsation massage in the ICU while he was being prepared for bypass surgery in 1994. (The nurses giving him the thigh massage were strikingly attractive young women, and my mother observed that my father seemed to be stimulated a little too much.) EECP was approved as a treatment for heart attacks in the ER the next year.

Does EECP have any effect on wheat and gluten problems?

EECP doesn't affect your reaction to wheat. However, your reaction to wheat, potatoes, and/or oats may affect inflammation in your belly flat. You may get belly-centered "swelling" when you eat these foods and that swelling places pressure on your heart. You may get some relief from heart problems when you reduce your consumption of these foods because your belly fat is not as inflamed. There are dozens of genes that determine the degree of your inflammatory reaction to these foods. This means that they affect different people in different degrees of severity. However, it also means that even a small change in consumption will have at least a small effect on how you feel. If you have full-blown celiac disease, which is a different problem, then you need to avoid wheat and other gluten grains in any amount.

Does EECP have any effect on sleep apnea?

No, but correcting sleep apnea can relieve pressure on the right side of your heart. EECP won't take the place of CPAP, but CPAP may have profound effects on heart health if you suffer sleep apnea.

Can people who have pacemakers or defibrillators have EECP?

Yes. If you have a pacemaker, that just means that EECP would pace itself to your pacemaker's rhythm. EECP has no effect on a pacemaker.

Are anticoagulants (blood thinners) an issue with EECP?

No. The pressure per square inch on your legs is so low that there is no risk of injury that could cause bleeding.

I have bad circulation in my legs (peripheral artery disease or venous insufficiency). Will EECP make the problem worse?

I have venous insufficiency myself. My symptoms improved after EECP (although I still opted to have a Venefit procedure about a month later). Venous insufficiency or PAD are not a barrier to EECP treatment, and they may improve during treatment. However, you may need more treatments to get the same effect because there is less circulation in the legs to generate a counter flow to the aorta.

How long do the benefits of EECP last?

Patients who have been followed by their doctors sustain cardiovascular benefits for three to five years. They may last longer, but patients have not been followed for more than five years in formal studies.

Can I repeat EECP?

Yes, if your doctor believes you can get even more benefit from another course of treatment, most insurance plans will let you have another 35 treatments three months after the most recent EECP treatment.

How do the results of EECP compare to angioplasty or stents?

If you are having a heart attack at the time you are admitted to a hospital, you will get percutaneous coronary intervention (angioplasty, stent, or both) or a bypass. If you are otherwise stable, however, EECP gets results as good or better than angioplasty or stents. "Results" include whether or not you need to go to the hospital again, whether or not you have a future heart attack or stroke, and whether or not you are still alive five years from now. It's not really a substitute for bypass surgery, but it is less risky that bypass surgery, and requires no recovery time.

Are there any ways in which EECP is better than angioplasty or stents?

There's a very important difference between EECP and typical treatments for coronary artery disease. Percutaneous coronary intervention (angioplasty or stents) just treats the symptoms of coronary artery disease. EECP induces changes in the physiology of the cardiovascular system that address the causes of atherosclerosis. EECP helps your blood vessels produce more nitric oxide. It opens arteries the same way nitroglycerin pills or nitrates (Imso, Imdur, Monoket, or isosorbide mononitrate) without risk of your body's becoming used to a medication. It reduces the production of endothelin, which makes blood vessels tight. EECP and also exercise programs (which take a lot longer and require a lot more effort) are cure rather than just treatment.

Can EECP dislodge cholesterol and cause a heart attack or stroke?

No. Your body's "plumbing" doesn't work that way. Blood always flows through the path of least resistance. Atherosclerosis increases resistance. EECP makes your blood flow away from areas of atherosclerosis to healthy blood vessels, and stimulates it to create more healthy blood vessels.

If I do EECP or start an exercise program and develop new collateral arteries, can I stop taking my statin for cholesterol?

No! Even if you have good cholesterol (a surprisingly large number of people who have heart attacks do) you need to continue your statin medication. It's not just for cholesterol. It's also to stop inflammation.

If you already have coronary artery disease, you almost certainly need a statin, a beta-blocker, an ACE inhibitor or an ACE-receptor blocker, and maybe nitrates and a sodium-channel blocker. Whether or not you take aspirin depends on which anticoagulant you take. If you are not on any anticoagulant, you will almost certainly be advised to take aspirin. Follow your doctor's orders on this. Don't try to change too many aspects of your treatment all at once.

You didn't mention weight loss in your diet chapter. Doesn't everybody who is on EECP need to lose weight?

Actually, most of the people I have met who were doing EECP were, unlike me, not in need of weight loss. You may experience some "water weight" loss as your circulation improves. However, EECP works independently of whether you are overweight, underweight, or just right.

Is EECP painful for people who have arthritis?

I have knee arthritis myself. I didn't have knee pain with EECP. That's because EECP places equal pressure on all sides of a joint, so it will not cause pain.

Are there any nutritional supplements that are helpful while I am doing EECP?

In the remote possibility you were protein-deficient (very few people are) L-arginine would help your body make nitric oxide to dilate arteries. However, it's extremely rare to need it.

Are there any supplements I should not take while I am doing EECP?

Acetyl-L-carnitine supplements seem to interfere with vascularization, as does green tea extract. Meat (the primary source of acetyl-L-carnitine in the diet) and green tea itself don't contain enough of the anti-angiogenic substances to cause problems.

What's that clip they keep putting on my finger during EECP?

Actually there are two "finger clips" used during EECP. At the beginning and end of every session the nurse or medical technician will measure your PulsOx. This device measures the percentage of oxygen compared to maximum that is in your bloodstream. During EECP treatment, the technician will use a different kind of sensor known as a *plethysmograph*. It collects data that are converted into a graphic representation, a finger *plethysmographic waveform*, that shows the flow of blood through your arteries. That's part of the "enhancement" that distinguishes EECP and ECP.

Plethysmography has its origins in Eastern Medicine, in which the doctor makes diagnoses through pulses. This device standardizes and quantifies "pulses" for easy interpretation and scientific validation.

Doesn't chelation therapy do the same thing as EECP?

I was taking chelation therapy that my hematologist (blood doctor) had prescribed for hemochromatosis (hereditary iron overload disease) while I was getting EECP, with the full knowledge of my cardiologist. However, I was getting a drug called deferasirox, not the EDTA that is often given as "chelation therapy" by naturopaths and other alternative practitioners. I was on a drug to lower iron levels, and it worked, but there was no expectation that this medication would affect my circulatory system.

I would like to be able to tell you that EDTA melts away cholesterol and makes your old arteries new again. Unfortunately, the Program to Assess Alternative Treatment Strategies to Achieve Cardiac Health (PATCH) Study just didn't find that it works. EDTA chelation may be helpful for diabetics who have heart disease, but it's not better than exercise or EECP. You won't get the $20,000 a month drug deferasirox unless you have high iron levels.

If EECP is so great why doesn't every doctor use it?

I'm editorializing, but I think the answer lies in economics. Medical care for heart health can be enormously expensive.

My grandmother had a heart attack in 1948. She was in the hospital for a few days, and sent home. Decades later, I found the hospital bill in my mother's papers.

Three days in the hospital had been billed at $23.75.

The cardiologist charged an additional $10.

Medications cost $1.25.

The terms were cash, payable at the time of discharge. My grandmother would not have insurance until the Medicare program started in 1965. But if three days in the hospital after you had heart attack only cost you $36, maybe even in 1948 you didn't have to worry about bankruptcy.

When I had a heart attack in 2017, my bill was a little bit more.

Thirty-six hours in the hospital were billed and percutaneous vascular intervention (a stent) cost $144,817.33.

The cardiologist billed an additional $57,310.21.

Medications, including my prescriptions for the first month after my heart attack, cost $18,745.90.

I had good insurance, and had already paid my deductible for the year before I had the heart attack. I just continued to pay my insurance premiums. My insurance company paid the rest.

The charges for my heart attack in 2017 were about 5,000 times higher than the charges for my grandmother in 1948. There's absolutely no doubt that my outcome was a lot more pleasant than hers. My grandma managed to live another 23 years after her heart attack. I don't know how long I will live after mine, but I do know that my quality of life is vastly better than my grandmother's. She suffered with stage II and stage III congestive heart failure, able to walk around her house but not much more, for decades. Three months after my heart attack in 2017, after 35 sessions of EECP, I was able to walk 800 meters in six minutes. That's the equivalent of running an 8-minute mile. If that's your personal best, you will never be a track star. But you're hardly an invalid, either.

So why doesn't every doctor recommend EECP? The answer is probably economics. My 35 hours of EECP resulted in a $4,480.00 charge, or a little over $125 a session. That has to cover (at least where I got my EECP) a staff of about 12, rent in a pricey office building, equipment, insurance, utilities, and a lot more. Plus my cardiologist supervises my treatment the entire seven weeks. Interventional cardiology makes more than a few millionaires. EECP never will. It struggles to pay the bills.

There was no grand conspiracy to hide EECP from the general public. Doctors are like the rest of us. They have to do the things that provide for themselves and their families. But they also have to follow standards of practice. One thing is for sure, when doctors offer EECP, it's not to make a lot of money. It's because it's the best alternative for their patients.

ENDNOTES

Introduction

1. Dr. Turner's testimony is online at http: // www.eecp.com/ testimonials.php, page 6. Portions of the testimony were confirmed from the Richmond Times Dispatch, September 9, 2009.

2. Molly's story is shared at http: //www.legacyheartcare.com/testimonials, and was verified with Legacy Heart Care staff.

3. Justine Reynolds' story is found at http: //www.eecp.com/ testimonials.php, page 11.

4. Dr. Whitaker records Chester's story at http: // whitakerwellness.com/therapies/eecp/eecp-therapy/.

5. Boren, C. Peyton Manning angrily denies report he used HGH, calls it "defamation." Washington Post, 27 December 2015.

6. Weinberger, D. Noninvasive treatment gives heart patients hope: Pulsating cuffs push blood to heart between beats, relieving pain from angina. Biz Journals Portland, 1 July 2005.

7. Liu L, Zhou S, Wu G, Zheng Z, Jin Y, Yang S, Zhan C, Fang D, Qian X. [Effects of external counterpulsation on the pulsatility of blood pressure in human subjects]. Sheng Wu Yi Xue Gong Cheng Xue Za Zhi. 2002 Sep; 19(3): 467-70. Chinese. PMID: 12557524.

Chapter 2. How Does EECP Work?

1. Akhtar M, Wu GF, Du ZM, Zheng ZS, Michaels AD. Effect of external counterpulsation on plasma nitric oxide and endothelin-1 levels.Am J Cardiol. 2006 Jul 1;98(1):28-30. Epub 2006 May 3.PMID: 16784915.

2. Dr. Kantrowitz's research is described in Braith RW, Casey DP, Beck DT. Enhanced External Counterpulsation for Ischemic Heart Disease: A Look Behind the Curtain.Exerc Sport Sci Rev. Author manuscript; available in PMC 2013 Jul 1.Published in final edited form as: Exerc Sport Sci Rev. 2012 Jul; 40(3): 145–152. doi: 10.1097/JES.0b013e318253de5e. PMCID: PMC3383356. See also: Birtwell WC, Giron F, Ruiz U, Norton RL, Soroff HS. The regional hemodynamic response to synchronous external pressure assist. Trans Am Soc Artif Intern Organs. 1970; 16: 462–5.

3. Arora RR, Chou TM, Jain D, Fleishman B, Crawford L, Mckiernan T, Nesto RW. The multicenter study of enhanced external counterpulsation (MUST-EECP): effect of EECP on exercise-induced myocardial ischemia and

anginal episodes. Journal of the American College of Cardiology. 1999; 33(7): 1833–40.

4. Stys TP, Lawson WE, Hui JC, Fleishman B, Manzo K, Strobeck JE, Tartaglia J, Ramasamy S, Suwita R, Zheng ZS, Liang H, Werner D. Effects of enhanced external counterpulsation on stress radionuclide coronary perfusion and exercise capacity in chronic stable angina pectoris. The American journal of cardiology. 2002; 89(7): 822–4.

5. Braith RW, Casey DP, Beck DT. Ibid.

6. Subramanian R, Nayar S, Meyyappan C, Ganesh N, Chandrakasu A, Nayar PG. Effect of Enhanced External Counter Pulsation Treatment on Aortic Blood Pressure, Arterial Stiffness and Ejection Fraction in Patients with Coronary Artery Disease. J Clin Diagn Res. 2016 Oct; 10(10): OC30-OC34. Epub 2016 Oct 1. PMID: 27891374.

7. Beck DT, Casey DP, Martin JS, Sardina PD, Braith RW. Enhanced external counterpulsation reduces indices of central blood pressure and myocardial oxygen demand in patients with left ventricular dysfunction. Clin Exp Pharmacol Physiol. 2015 Apr; 42(4): 315-20. doi: 10.1111/1440-1681.12367. PMID: 25676084.

8. Martin JS, Beck DT, Braith RW. Peripheral resistance artery blood flow in subjects with abnormal glucose tolerance is improved following enhanced external counterpulsation therapy. Appl Physiol Nutr Metab. 2014 May; 39(5): 596-9. doi: 10.1139/apnm-2013-0497. Epub 2013 PMID: 24766247.

9. Martin JS, Braith RW. Anti-inflammatory effects of enhanced external counterpulsation in subjects with abnormal glucose tolerance.Appl Physiol Nutr Metab. 2012

Dec; 37(6): 1251-5. doi: 10.1139/h2012-112. Epub 2012 Oct 11. PMID: 23057577.

10. Lawson WE, Hui JC, Kennard ED, Soran O, McCullough PA, Kelsey SF; IEPR Investigators. Effect of enhanced external counterpulsation on medically refractory angina patients with erectile dysfunction. Int J Clin Pract. 2007 May; 61(5): 757-62. PMID: 17493089.

11. May O, Søgaard HJ. Enhanced External Counterpulsation Is an Effective Treatment for Depression in Patients With Refractory Angina Pectoris. Prim Care Companion CNS Disord. 2015 Aug 20; 17(4). doi: 10.4088/PCC.14m01748. eCollection 2015. PMID: 26693035.

12. Levenson J, Simon A, Megnien JL, Chironi G, Gariepy J, Pernollet MG, Craiem D, Iliou MC. Effects of enhanced external counterpulsation on carotid circulation in patients with coronary artery disease. Cardiology. 2007; 108(2): 104-10. Epub 2006 Sep 29. PMID: 17008798.

Chapter 3. What Else Can EECP Do for You?

1. Myhre LG, Muir I, Schutz RW, Rantala B, Thigpen T. Enhanced external counterpulsation for improving athletic performance. Paper presented at: Experimental Biology 2004 (2004) April 17–21, Washington, DC.

2. Werner D, Trägner P, Wawer A, Porst H, Daniel WG, Gross P. Enhanced external counterpulsation: a new technique to augment renal function in liver cirrhosis. Nephrol Dial Transplant. 2005 May; 20(5): 920-6. Epub 2005 Mar 23. PMID: 15788437.

3. Sardina PD, Martin JS, Avery JC, Braith RW. Enhanced external counterpulsation (EECP) improves biomarkers of glycemic control in patients with non-insulin-dependent type II diabetes mellitus for up to 3 months following treatment. Acta Diabetol. 2016 Oct; 53(5): 745-52. doi: 10.1007/s00592-016-0866-9. Epub 2016 May 14. PMID: 27179825.

4. Sardina PD, Martin JS, Dzieza WK, Braith RW. Enhanced external counterpulsation (EECP) decreases advanced glycation end products and proinflammatory cytokines in patients with non-insulin-dependent type II diabetes mellitus for up to 6 months following treatment. Acta Diabetol. 2016 Oct; 53(5): 753-60. doi: 10.1007/s00592-016-0869-6. Epub 2016 Jun 9. PMID: 27278477.

5. Lawson WE, Hui JC, Kennard ED, Soran O, McCullough PA, Kelsey SF; IEPR Investigators. Effect of enhanced external counterpulsation on medically refractory angina patients with erectile dysfunction. Int J Clin Pract. 2007 May; 61(5): 757-62. PMID: 17493089.

6. Lawson WE, Hui JC, Kennard ED, Kelsey SF, Michaels AD, Soran O; International Enhanced External Counterpulsation Patient Registry Investigators. Two-year outcomes in patients with mild refractory angina treated with enhanced external counterpulsation. Clin Cardiol. 2006 Feb; 29(2): 69-73. PMID: 16506642.

7. Rajaram SS, Rudzinskiy P, Walters AS. Enhanced external counter pulsation (EECP) for restless legs syndrome (RLS): preliminary negative results in a parallel double-blind study. Sleep Med. 2006 Jun; 7(4): 390-1. Epub 2006 May 19. PMID: 16713348.

Chapter 4. Can Everybody Get EECP?

1. Michaels AD, Accad M, Ports TA, Grossman W. Left ventricular systolic unloading and augmentation of intracoronary pressure and Doppler flow during enhanced external counterpulsation. Circulation. 2002 Sep 3; 106(10): 1237-42. PMID: 12208799.

2. Jørgensen PG, Lindberg JA, May O. Toxic shock syndrome: A rare complication to enhanced external counterpulsation. Can J Cardiol. 2010 Dec; 26(10): e351-2. PMID: 21165367.

Chapter 5: How to Be Sure You Succeed with EECP

1. Zheng ZS, Li TM, Kambie H, Chen GH, Yu LQ, Cai SR, Zhan CY,Chen YC, Wo SX, Chen GW: Sequential external counterpulsation(SECP) in China. Transactions of the American Society for Arti-ficial Internal Organs 1983; 29: 599–603.

2. Wu GF, Zheng OS, Zheng ZS, Zhang MQ, Lawson WE, Hui JCK: A neurohormonal mechanism for the effectiveness of enhanced external counterpulsation (abstr 4390). Circulation 1999; 100(suppl1): I-832.

3. Braverman DL, Wechsler B. Enhanced External Counterpulsation and Functional Improvement in Octogenarians with Ischemic Heart Disease. Arch Phys Med Rehab. 84 (2003): 10-23.

4. Linnemeier G, Michaels AD, Soran O, Kennard ED; International Enhanced External Counterpulsation Patient Registry Investigators. Enhanced external counterpulsation

in the management of angina in the elderly. Am J Geriatr Cardiol. 2003 Mar-Apr; 12(2): 90-4; quiz 94-6. PMID: 12624578.

5. Malenka DJ, O'Rourke D, Miller MA, Hearne MJ, Shubrooks S, Kellett MA Jr, Robb JF, O'Meara JR, VerLee P, Bradley WA, Wennberg D, Ryan T Jr, Vaitkus PT, Hettleman B, Watkins MW, McGrath PD, O'Connor GT. Cause of in-hospital death in 12,232 consecutive patients undergoing percutaneous transluminal coronary angioplasty. The Northern New England Cardiovascular Disease Study Group. Am Heart J. 1999 Apr; 137(4 Pt 1): 632-8.

6. Vaccarino V, Lin ZQ, Kasl SV, Mattera JA, Roumanis SA, Abramson JL, Krumholz HM. Sex differences in health status after coronary artery bypass surgery. Circulation. 2003 Nov 25; 108(21): 2642-7. Epub 2003 Nov 3. PMID: 14597590.

7. Efstratiadis S, Kennard ED, Kelsey SF, Michaels AD; International EECP Patient Registry-2 Investigators.. Passive tobacco exposure may impair symptomatic improvement in patients with chronic angina undergoing enhanced external counterpulsation. BMC Cardiovasc Disord. 2008 Sep 17; 8: 23. doi: 10.1186/1471-2261-8-23.

PMID: 18798998.

8. May O, Søgaard HJ. Enhanced External Counterpulsation Is an Effective Treatment for Depression in Patients With Refractory Angina Pectoris. Prim Care Companion CNS Disord. 2015 Aug 20; 17(4). doi: 10.4088/PCC.14m01748. eCollection 2015. PMID: 26693035.

9. Kozdağ G, Işeri P, Gökçe G, Ertaş G, Aygün F, Kutlu A, Hebert K, Ural D. Treatment with enhanced external counterpulsation improves cognitive functions in chronic heart failure patients. Turk Kardiyol Dern Ars. 2013 Jul; 41(5) : 418-28. doi: 10.5543/ tkda.2013.24366. PMID: 23917007.

10. Martin JS, Beck DT, Aranda JM Jr, Braith RW. Enhanced external counterpulsation improves peripheral artery function and glucose tolerance in subjects with abnormal glucose tolerance. J Appl Physiol (1985). 2012 Mar; 112(5): 868-76. doi: 10.1152/ japplphysiol.01336.2011. Epub 2011 Dec 22. PMID: 22194326.

11. Tarpgaard Jørgensen M, Gerdes C, May O. Prinzmetal's variant angina is effectively treated with enhanced external counterpulsation. Acta Cardiol. 2010 Apr; 65(2): 265-7. PMID: 20458840.

12 Fitzgerald CP, Lawson WE, Hui JC, Kennard ED; IEPR Investigators. Enhanced external counterpulsation as initial revascularization treatment for angina refractory to medical therapy. Cardiology. 2003; 100(3): 129-35.

PMID: 14631133.

13. Lawson WE, Hui JC, Guo T, Burger L, Cohn PF. Prior revascularization increases the effectiveness of enhanced external counterpulsation. Clin Cardiol. 1998 Nov; 21(11): 841-4. PMID: 9825198.

Chapter 6. Is There an EECP Diet?

1. Asgary S, Afshani MR, Sahebkar A, Keshvari M, Taheri M, Jahanian E, Rafieian-Kopaei M, Malekian F, Sarrafzadegan N. Improvement of hypertension,

endothelial function and systemic inflammation following short-term supplementation with red beet (Beta vulgaris L.) juice: a randomized crossover pilot study. J Hum Hypertens. 2016 Oct; 30(10): 627-32. doi: 10.1038/jhh.2016.34. Epub 2016 Jun 9. PMID: 27278926.

2. Nyakayiru J, Jonvik KL, Trommelen J, Pinckaers PJ, Senden JM, van Loon LJ, Verdijk LB. Beetroot Juice Supplementation Improves High-Intensity Intermittent Type Exercise Performance in Trained Soccer Players. Nutrients. 2017 Mar 22; 9(3). pii: E314. doi: 10.3390/nu9030314.

PMID: 28327503.

3. Larsen FJ, Weitzberg E, Lundberg JO, Ekblom B. Effects of dietary nitrate on oxygen cost during exercise. Acta Physiol (Oxf). 2007 Sep; 191(1): 59-66. Epub 2007 Jul 17. PMID: 17635415.

4. Larsen FJ, Schiffer TA, Borniquel S, Sahlin K, Ekblom B, Lundberg JO, Weitzberg E. Dietary inorganic nitrate improves mitochondrial efficiency in humans.Cell Metab. 2011 Feb 2; 13(2): 149-59. doi: 10.1016/ j.cmet.2011.01.004 .PMID: 21284982.

5. Esser D, Oosterink E, op 't Roodt J, Henry RM, Stehouwer CD, Müller M, Afman LA. Vascular and inflammatory high fat meal responses in young healthy men; a discriminative role of IL-8 observed in a randomized trial.

PLoS One. 2013; 8(2): e53474. doi: 10.1371/journal.pone.0053474. Epub 2013 Feb 6. PMID: 23405070.

6. Casas R, Urpi-Sardà M, Sacanella E, Arranz S, Corella D, Castañer O, Lamuela-Raventós RM, Salas-Salvadó J,

Lapetra J, Portillo MP, Estruch R. Anti-Inflammatory Effects of the Mediterranean Diet in the Early and Late Stages of Atheroma Plaque Development. Mediators Inflamm. 2017; 2017: 3674390. doi: 10.1155/2017/3674390. Epub 2017 Apr 18. PMID: 28484308.

Chapter 7. What Do You Do After EECP?

1. For instance, these two studies:

Cannon CP, Weintraub WS, Demopoulos LA, Vicari R, Frey MJ, Lakkis N: Comparison of early invasive and conservative strategies in patients with unstable coronary syndromes treated with the glycoprotein IIb/IIIa inhibitor tirofiban. N Engl J Med. 2001, 344: 1879-1887. 10.1056/NEJM200106213442501.

Lagerqvist B, Husted S, Kontny F, Stshle E, Swahn E, Wallentin L: 5-year outcomes in the FRISC-II randomised trial of an invasive versus a non-invasive strategy in non-ST-elevation acute coronary syndrome: a follow-up study. Lancet. 2006, 368: 998-1004. 10.1016/S0140-6736(06)69416-6.

2. For instance, these four studies:

Boden WE, O'Rourke RA, Teo KK, Hartigan PM, Maron DJ, Kostuk WJ: Optimal medical therapy with or without PCI for stable coronary disease. N Engl J Med. 2007, 356: 1503-1516. 10.1056/NEJMoa070829.

Boden WE, O'Rourke RA, Teo KK, Maron DJ, Hartigan PM, Sedlis SP: Impact of optimal medical therapy with or without percutaneous coronary intervention on long-term cardiovascular end points in patients with stable coronary artery disease (from the COURAGE trial). Am J Cardiol. 2009, 104: 1-4. 10.1016/j.amjcard.2009.02.059

Frye RL, August P, Brooks MM, Hardison RM, Kelsey SF, MacGregor JM: A randomized trial of therapies for type 2 diabetes and coronary artery disease. N Engl J Med. 2009, 360: 2503-2515.

Sedlis SP, Jurkovitz CT, Hartigan PM, Goldfarb DS, Lorin JD, Dada M: Optimal medical therapy with or without percutaneous coronary intervention for patients with stable coronary artery disease and chronic kidney disease. Am J Cardiol. 2009, 104: 1647-1653. 10.1016/j.amjcard.2009.07.043.

3. Möbius-Winkler S, Uhlemann M, Adams V, Sandri M, Erbs S, Lenk K, Mangner N, Mueller U, Adam J, Grunze M, Brunner S, Hilberg T, Mende M, Linke AP, Schuler G. Coronary Collateral Growth Induced by Physical Exercise: Results of the Impact of Intensive Exercise Training on Coronary Collateral Circulation in Patients With Stable Coronary Artery Disease (EXCITE) Trial.Circulation. 2016 Apr 12; 133(15): 1438-48; discussion 1448. doi: 10.1161/CIRCULATIONAHA.115.016442. Epub 2016 Mar 15. PMID: 26979085.

4. Figueroa A, Jaime SJ, Alvarez-Alvarado S. Whole-body vibration as a potential countermeasure for dynapenia and arterial stiffness. Integr Med Res. 2016 Sep; 5(3): 204-211. doi: 10.1016/j.imr.2016.06.004. Epub 2016 Jun 18. Review. PMID: 28462119.

5. Elfering A, Burger C, Schade V, Radlinger L. Stochastic resonance whole body vibration increases perceived muscle relaxation but not cardiovascular activation: A randomized

controlled trial. World J Orthop. 2016 Nov 18; 7(11): 758-765. eCollection 2016 Nov 18. PMID: 27900274.

6. Verschueren SM, Roelants M, Delecluse C, Swinnen S, Vanderschueren D, Boonen S. Effect of 6-month whole body vibration training on hip density, muscle strength, and postural control in postmenopausal women: a randomized controlled pilot study. J Bone Miner Res. 2004; 19: 352–359

7. Fjeldstad C, Palmer IJ, Bemben MG, Bemben DA. Whole-body vibration augments resistance training effects on body composition in postmenopausal women. Maturitas. 2009; 63: 79–83.

8. Nakamura H, Okazawa T, Nagase H, Yoshida M, Ariizumi M, Okada A. Change in digital blood flow with simultaneous reduction in plasma endothelin induced by hand-arm vibration. Int Arch Occup Environ Health. 1996; 68: 115–119.

9. Maloney-Hinds C, Petrofsky JS, Zimmerman G, Hessinger DA. The role of nitric oxide in skin blood flow increases due to vibration in healthy adults and adults with type 2 diabetes. Diabetes Technol Ther. 2009; 11: 39–43.

10. Supa'at I, Zakaria Z, Maskon O, Aminuddin A, Nordin NA. Effects of Swedish massage therapy on blood pressure, heart rate, and inflammatory markers in hypertensive women. Evid Based Complement Alternat Med. 2013; 2013: 171852. doi: 10.1155/2013/171852. Epub 2013 Aug 18. PMID: 24023571.

11. Givi M. Durability of effect of massage therapy on blood pressure. Int J Prev Med. 2013 May; 4(5): 511-6. PMID: 23930160.

12. Nivethitha L, Mooventhan A, Manjunath NK. Effects of Various Prāṇāyāma on Cardiovascular and Autonomic Variables. Anc Sci Life. 2016 Oct-Dec; 36(2): 72-77. doi: 10.4103/asl.ASL_178_16. Review. PMID: 28446827.

13. Bhavanani AB, Madanmohan, Sanjay Z, Basavaraddi IV. Immediate cardiovascular effects of pranava pranayama in hypertensive patients. Indian J Physiol Pharmacol. 2012; 56: 273–8.

14. Bhavanani AB, Sanjay Z, Madanmohan Immediate effect of sukha pranayama on cardiovascular variables in patients of hypertension. Int J Yoga Therap. 2011; 21: 73–6.

15. Pohl T, Wustmann K, Zbinden S, Windecker S, Mehta H, Meier B: Exercise-induced human coronary collateral function: quantitative assessment during acute coronary occlusions. Cardiology. 2003, 100: 53-60. 10.1159/000073039.

16. Murphy M, Nevill A, Neville C, Biddle S, Hardman A. Accumulating brisk walking for fitness, cardiovascular risk, and psychological health. Med Sci Sports Exerc. 2002 Sep; 34(9): 1468-74. PMID: 12218740.

17. Nualnim N, Parkhurst K, Dhindsa M, Tarumi T, Vavrek J, Tanaka H. Effects of swimming training on blood pressure and vascular function in adults > 50 years of age. Am J Cardiol. 2012 Apr 1; 109(7): 1005-10. doi: 10.1016/j.amjcard.2011.11.029. Epub 2012 Jan 11. PMID: 22244035.

18. Hopkins DR, Murrah B, Hoeger WW, Rhodes RC. Effect of low-impact aerobic dance on the functional fitness of elderly women. Gerontologist. 1990 Apr; 30(2): 189-92. PMID: 2347499.

19. Yeh GY, McCarthy EP, Wayne PM, Stevenson LW, Wood MJ, Forman D, Davis RB, Phillips RS. Tai chi exercise in patients with chronic heart failure: a randomized clinical trial. Arch Intern Med. 2011 Apr 25; 171(8): 750-7. doi: 10.1001/ archinternmed.2011.150. PMID: 21518942.

20. Damodaran A, Malathi A, Patil N, Shah N, Suryavansihi, Marathe S. Therapeutic potential of yoga practices in modifying cardiovascular risk profile in middle aged men and women. J Assoc Physicians India. 2002 May; 50(5): 633-40. PMID: 12186115.

21. Parker ND, Hunter GR, Treuth MS, Kekes-Szabo T, Kell SH, Weinsier R, White M. Effects of strength training on cardiovascular responses during a submaximal walk and a weight-loaded walking test in older females. J Cardiopulm Rehabil. 1996 Jan-Feb; 16(1): 56-62. PMID: 8907443.

GLOSSARY

Abdominal aortic aneurysm (AAA). A sac-like expansion of abdominal aorta due to a weakness in the artery wall.

Angina (angina pectoris). A collection of symptoms that the heart is not receiving enough blood. Commonly described as chest pain, although in older people it is often experienced as pressure rather than pain, and the pain can be referred to other parts of the body, not just the left arm, the chin, or the neck.

Anginal equivalents. Symptoms other than pain that indicate that the heart is not getting enough oxygen. Can include shortness of breath, fatigue, heartburn, vomiting, nausea, or palpitations, as well as unusual pain or pressure in the shoulders, shoulder blades, or legs.

Angiogenesis. The growth of new blood vessels, including those that grow around blockages.

Angiogram. Clinical report of the results of a coronary catheterization or angiography.

Angiography. See Cardiac catheterization.

Angioplasty. Procedure in which a balloon is inserted into the center of an artery and inflated to push the blockage to the sides of the artery. Also called percutaneous transluminal coronary angioplasty or PTCA.

Anticoagulant. A medication to prevent blood clotting.

Aorta. The largest blood vessel in the body. All the output of the left ventricle travels through the aorta after it leaves the heart.

Aortic insufficiency (AI). Also known as aortic regurgitation (AR). A failure or leakage of the valves that allow the aorta to close with the result that blood flows back into the left ventricle (regurgitation) rather than through the aorta and into the coronary arteries.

Aortic valve. The valve between the left ventricle of the heart and the aorta. Closure of this valve signals the end of systole (contraction of the heart) and the beginning of diastole (relaxation of the heart).

Arrhythmia. Irregular heartbeat.

Arteries. Blood vessels that carry oxygenated blood away from the heart and throughout the body.

Atherosclerosis. Also known as "hardening of the arteries," the process of calcification of cholesterol, white blood cells, and other matter that makes specific sites in arteries inflexible and later clogged.

Atrial fibrillation. Also known as "A-fib," a condition of disturbed electrical conduction in the upper chambers of the heart that results in an irregular heart rhythm and a tendency to form blood clots.

Atrium. One of the upper chambers of the heart (plural: atria).

Augmentation. In ECP and EECP, an increase in diastolic blood pressure (due to the application of pressure in cuffs placed on the legs and waist) that results in reversal of blood flow from the heart in a "wave" from the legs up.

Autoimmune. Refers to attacks by the immune system on the body's own tissues.

Blood pressure. The pressure of blood against artery walls, or the pressure exerted by the heart as it pumps blood.

BPM (or bpm). Beats per minute, referring to heartbeat.

B-type natriuretic peptide. Also known as plasma brain-type natriuretic peptide, a substance released by the ventricles of the heart in response to changes in blood pressure in congestive heart failure.

Bypass surgery, CABG. See Coronary artery bypass graft.

CAD. *See* Coronary artery disease.

Cardiac. Relating to the heart.

Cardiac catheterization. A procedure in which a long, thin tube (catheter) is inserted through a small incision into an artery to deliver dye to the heart that allows x-rays of the heart to be taken so that its structures and blood vessels are visible.

Cardiac cycle. Sequence of events from one heartbeat to the next. See also Diastole and Systole.

Cardiac output. The amount of oxygenated blood sent by the heart to the arteries in one minute (in adults, usually four to six liters).

Cardiomyopathy. A condition of tissue damage in the heart in which it may lack pumping power (dilated cardiomyopathy), lack the ability to fill with blood (restricted cardiomyopathy), or be thickened (hypertrophic cardiomyopathy).

Cardiovascular disease. A group of diseases affecting the heart and blood vessels including hypertension, coronary artery disease, and peripheral vascular disease.

CAT scan. *See* Computed tomography.

Cerebral vascular accident (CVA). An injury to the brain caused by interruption of block flow (ischemia) or bleeding (hemorrhage), also known as a stroke.

CHD. Coronary heart disease.

CHF. Congestive heart failure.

Claudication. A symptom of peripheral vascular disease in which exercise (walking, for example) results in pain. Pain caused by exertion tends to indicate an arterial problem, while pain caused by standing tends to indicate a venous problem.

Collateral blood vessels. Small blood vessels that develop over time in response to backward flow of blood due to an obstruction. These blood vessels reroute blood around a blockage. EECP is a method of accelerating the growth of collateral blood vessels.

Computed tomography (CAT scan, CT scan). A combination of X-ray and computer technology that creates cross-sectional images of structures and tissues in the body.

Congestive heart failure. A condition in which the heart muscle is too weak to pump blood throughout the entire body, almost always causing shortness of breath and swelling in the feet and legs.

Coronary. Relating to the heart.

Coronary artery bypass graft (CABG). Also known as bypass surgery or open-heart surgery, a procedure using a vein or artery to create a new path for blood to flow around a blockage.

Coronary artery disease (CAD). A condition of reduced flexibility and obstruction of an artery providing blood to the heart or directing blood away from the heart.

Coronary heart disease (CHD). A condition of reduced blood flow to the heart, usually due to atherosclerosis.

Coumadin. The North American brand name for warfarin, an anticoagulant that acts by interfering with vitamin K-1.

C-reactive protein (C-RP). A protein produced by the liver during incidents of acute inflammation, such as coronary artery disease.

CT scan. Computed tomography.

Deep vein thrombosis (DVT). A clot in a deep vein in the legs, or sometimes in the pelvis or arms.

Diabetes. A condition in which the body does not respond to or does not produce insulin properly, resulting in elevated blood sugar levels.

Diastole. The resting phase of the cardiac cycle, during which the heart receives 70 to 80 percent of its blood supply. Diastole begins when the aortic valve closes.

Diastolic augmentation. A measure of the flow of blood in the arteries of the heart.

Diastolic blood pressure. The lowest blood pressure between heartbeats.

Diuresis. The process by which the body relieves itself of excess fluid.

Diuretic. A medication that increases diuresis.

Doppler ultrasound (or just "ultrasound"). A noninvasive method of measuring blood flow through and around the heart.

DVT. See Deep vein thrombosis.

ECG. Electrocardiogram, also known as EKG.

Echocardiogram, also known as "echo." A procedure that uses ultrasound to produce a moving picture outline of the heart's valves and chambers.

Edema. Swelling due to accumulation of excessive fluid. Usually occurs in the feet or hands, but may occur in the abdomen.

ECP. Extracorporeal counterpulsation therapy, a method of encouraging the growth of collateral blood vessels.

EECP. Enhanced extracorporeal counterpuslation therapy, a method of encouraging the growth of collateral blood vessels augmented by technology patented by a company called Vasotech.

Ejection fraction. The ratio of blood that is pumped with each beat of the heart to the blood that fills the heart between beats, usually expressed as percent.

Electrocardiogram (also known as ECG or EKG). A record of the heart's electrical activity.

Embolus. A blood clot that travels through the bloodstream (plural: emboli).

Endothelial cells. Cells that line blood vessels and play a role in regulating blood flow.

Endothelin (ET-1). A substance released by endothelial cells that causes blood vessels to constrict and raises blood pressure.

Enhanced external counterpulsation therapy (EECP). A patented procedure that non-invasively increases circulation to the heart between heart beats to encourage the accelerated formation of collateral blood vessels while reducing the production of ET-1 and relieving the work load of the heart. EECP is the application of "enhanced" technology patented by Vasotech, while ECP is other applications of very similar technique. Nearly all research studies published in English involve EECP, not ECP ("external counterpulsation therapy," without the enhancements provided by Vasotech).

Heart attack. See Myocardial infarction.

Heart disease. A generic term commonly including all diseases of the heart.

Heart failure. A condition in which the heart is too weak to pump enough blood for the body's needs.

Hypertension, sometimes noted as HTN. High blood pressure.

Implantable cardioverter defibrillator (ICD), generally referred to as a "defibrillator." Surgically implanted electronic device that constantly monitors heart rate and rhythm, delivering an electric shock when certain kinds of potentially dangerous arrhythmias occur. No defibrillator can be calibrated to correct every kind of potentially dangerous arrhythmia.

International normalized ratio (INR). A standard measurement of coagulation of the blood, used to choose the appropriate dosage of anticoagulants.

Ischemia. A deficiency of blood supply and oxygen delivery, so that oxygen demand of a tissue is greater than its supply.

Myocardial. Referring to the heart muscle.

Myocardial infarction (MI). Commonly termed a "heart attack," the destruction of areas of heart muscle after deprivation of blood supply. The actual destruction of the muscle may only occur when its oxygen supply is restored, see Reperfusion injury.

Myocardial perfusion. The pattern of blood flow through heart muscle.

Myocardium. The heart muscle.

Nitric oxide (NO). A substance released by endothelial cells that causes a blood vessel to dilate and relax.

Occlusion. Blockage.

Open-heart surgery. See *Coronary artery bypass graft.*

Pacemaker. A surgically implanted electronic device that sends electrical signals to the heart muscles to maintain a steady heart rhythm.

Percutaneous coronary intervention (PCI). An invasive, surgical procedure in which a small incision is made in peripheral artery, usually in the groin or in the arm, and a catheter is inserted to be threaded to a blockage elsewhere in the body. Angioplasty, angiography, and stent placements are performed with this procedure.

Peripheral vascular disease (PVD). Diseases of blood vessels outside the heart and brain, most commonly narrowing of the arteries that supply blood to the feet and legs.

PET scan. See Positron emission tomography.

Plaque. Deposits of calcium, cholesterol, and white blood cells that accumulate in the linings of arteries and impede blood flow.

Plethysmograph. The sensor put on your finger during EECP treatment that creates a waveform that represents patterns in your circulation. This is not the PulsOx sensor that is used at the beginning and end of a session to make sure your oxygen levels are adequate.

Positron emission tomography (PET scan). Nuclear scan that provides a three-dimensional picture of blood flow through the coronary arteries.

Premature ventricular contraction (PVC). Condition in which the ventricles contract before they are supposed to.

PTCA. Percutaneous transluminal coronary angioplasty. See Angioplasty.

Refractory angina. Persistent angina in people who cannot receive further surgery and cannot be given more medication.

Restenosis. Narrowing or closing of an artery previously opened by a PCI, such as angioplasty or a stent.

Silent ischemia. Inadequate blood supply without symptoms.

Stable angina. Heart-related pain that occurs predictably after exertion and lasts less than 30 minutes, usually relieved with nitroglycerin. May persist for years.

Stenosis. Restriction or narrowing of a blood vessel, reducing blood flow.

Stent. A metal device inserted into an artery and expanded to increase blood flow.

Stress test. A procedure to see how well the heart works, either under conditions of exercise or after injection of a chemical.

Stroke. See *Cerebral vascular accident.*

Stroke volume. The amount of blood the heart pumps in one beat.

Systemic vascular resistance (SVR). Resistance to the flow of blood out the left ventricle and into the rest of the body.

Systole. The "pumping" or contraction phase of heart beat.

Systolic. The highest blood pressure measured in an artery, as the heart contracts.

Thrombophlebitis. The inflammation of a vein, usually in connection with a blood clot, usually in the legs.

Thrombus. A blood clot.

Ultrasound. A non-invasive diagnostic method using high-frequency sound waves to create visual images of soft tissues in the body.

Unstable angina. Angina that occurs even without exercise or at unpredictable times.

Vascular endothelial growth factor (VEGF). Hormone that promotes the growth of new blood vessels.

Vasoconstriction. Narrowing of a blood vessel, causing reduced blood flow and higher pressure.

Vasoconstrictor. A medication that causes constriction of a blood vessel, reducing blood flow through the vessel.

Vasodilator. A medication that causes dilation or relaxation of a blood vessel, increasing blood flow through the vessel.

Vein. Blood vessel that conducts blood back to the heart.

Ventricle. One of the lower chambers of the heart.

WHERE TO GET EECP IN THE USA

Not every state in the United States has a provider of EECP, but sometimes there are center in nearby states. To facilitate locating EECP providers across state lines, this section lists their offices by zip codes.

Every effort has been made to ensure that the listings here are up to date, but it's always best to call ahead—and you will need a doctor's referral before treatment to get insurance reimbursement. Providers listed here were affiliated with Vasotech ® at the time this book was written (April 2017). Even better, let your cardiologist handle the referrals.

01854

Lowell General Hospital
295 Varnum Avenue
Lowell, MA 1854
(978) 934-8238

06040

Eastern CT Cardiology Association, LLC
43 West Middle Turnpike
Manchester, CT 06040
(860) 647-9494
www.eecallc.com

06117

Hartford Cardiology Group
345 North Main Street, First Floor
West Hartford, CT 06117
(860) 547-1489
www.hartfordcardiology.com

07031

North Arlington Cardiology Associates, PA
62 Ridge Road
North Arlington, NJ 7031
(201) 991-8565

07093

Luis A. Gonzalez, MD
325 60th Street, PO Box 277
West New York, NJ 7093
(201) 868-6626

07306

The Heart Center
600 Pavonia Avenue
Jersey City, NJ 7306
(201) 216-3060

07656

The Heart Center at Glenpointe

400 Frank W. Burr Blvd. 2nd Fl
Teaneck, NJ 07666
(201) 907-0442

07666

The Heart Center at Glenpointe
400 Frank W. Burr Blvd. 2nd Fl
Teaneck, NJ 07666
(201) 907-0442

08057

Virtua
401 Young Avenue, #275
Moorestown, NJ 08057
(856) 234-3332

08080

Cardiovascular Associates of Delaware Valley
570 Egg Harbor Road Suite B-1
Sewell, NJ 8080
(856) 582-2000

08360

Cumberland Professional Campus
1051 West Sherman Avenue
Vineland, NJ 08360
(856) 691-8070

10001

New York Cardiovascular Associates, PLLC
275 Seventh Avenue, Suite 302
New York, NY 10001
(646) 660-9999

10013

Michael Poon, MD
70 Bowery, Suite 303
New York, NY 10013
(212) 925-4088

10605

Joseph Tartaglia, MD
311 North Street, Suite 301
White Plains, NY 10605
(914) 946-3388

10605

University Physicians - Stony Brook
200 Motor Pkwy., Suite C
Hauppauge, NY 11788
(631) 444-8420

11042

NYU Langone Long Island Cardiac Care
1 Hollow Lane
Lake Success, NY 11042
(516) 869-5400

11201

Sarath Reddy, MD
240 Willoughby Street, Suite 11E
Brooklyn, NY 11201
(718) 250-8627

11201

Jasty & Manvar, MD Cardiologist
240 Willoughby Street, 10 F
Brooklyn , NY 11201

(718) 783-7001

11422
Queens Heart Institute, Strong Health Medical, PC
234-36 Merrick Blvd.
Laurelton, NY 11422
(718) 949-9400

11548
St. Francis Hospital
101 Northern Blvd., CHF Dept.
Greenvale, NY 11548
(516) 629-2090

11758
Cardiology & Internal Medicine of Long Island
510 Hicksville Road
Massapequa, NY 11758
(516) 795-2626

11788
University Physicians - Stony Brook
200 Motor Pkwy., Suite C
Hauppauge, NY 11788
(631) 444-8420

13676
Canton Potsdam Hospital
50 Leroy Street
Potsdam, NY 13676
(315) 265-3300
www.cphospital.org

17403
Apple Hill Medical Center
25 Monument Road, Suite 199, Entrance C
York, PA 17403
(717) 741-8280

19610
Cardiology Associates of West Reading
1320 Brodcasting Road
Wyomissing, PA 19610
(610) 375-6565

20850
Shady Grove Adventist Cardiopulmonary Rehab &
EECP® Center
9715 Medical Center Drive, Suite 130
Rockville, MD 20850
(240) 826-6662

21601
Shore Health Systems
219 S. Washington Street
Easton, MD 21601
(410) 822-1000

22031
EECP® Center of Northern Virginia
3023 Hamaker Court, Suite 100
Fairfax, VA 22031
(703) 641-9161

22401
Mary Washington Hospital
1021B Sam Perry Blvd Ste 240

Fredericksburg, VA 22401
(540) 741-1348

22601

Winchester Medical Center VH
1840 Amherst St.
Winchester, VA 22601
(540) 536-0517

24501

Stroobants Cardiovascular Center
2410 Atherholt Rd.
Lynchburg, VA 24501
(434) 200-5252

25301

EECP® of W. VA
1208 Kanawha Blvd. E.
Charleston, WV 25301
(304) 414-0090

25704

Veterans Affairs Medical Center
1540 Spring Valley Drive
Huntington, WV 25704
(304) 429-6755

27103

Forsyth Medical Center
3333 Silas Creek Parkway
Winston-Salem, NC 27103
(336) 718-6199

27710

Duke University Medical Center South
40 Duke Medicine Cir
Durham, NC 27710
(919) 681-6234

28211

Legacy Heart Care
300 Billingsley Rd. Suite 101
Charlotte, NC 28211
(704) 334-1401
www.legacyheartcare.com

28304

Cape Fear Cardiology Associates
3634 Cape Center Drive
Fayetteville, NC 28304
(910) 485-6470

28304

Carolina Cardiology
3656 Cape Center Drive
Fayetteville, NC 28304
(910) 221-1206

28358

Duke: Southeastern Regional Medical Center
300 West 27th Street
Lumberton, NC 28358
(910) 671-6619

30546

Health in Harmony
1220 Chatuge Circle

Hiawassee, GA 30546
(706) 896-9442

31792
Cardiology Consultants of South Georgia
100 Mimosa Dr., 2nd Floor
Thomasville, GA 31792
(229) 551-0083

32034
Baptist Heart Specialists
1340 South 18th St., Bldg A - Ste 202
Fernandina Beach, FL 32034
(904) 261-9786

32216
Drs. Baker & Gilmour, MD, PA
3550 University Blvd, Suite 302
Jacksonville, FL 32216
(904) 733-4444

32401
Northwest Florida Cardiovascular Associates
801 East 6th Street, Suite 504
Panama City, FL 32401
(850) 769-0329

33069
Heart Group of Broward
150 SW 12th Ave., Suite 480
Pompano Beach, FL 33069
(954) 565-5807

33145

Miami Heart Center
1990 SW 27th Avenue, 2nd Floor
Miami, FL 33145
(305) 442-1159

33172
Institute for Cardiovascular Disease, PA
2301 NW 87th Ave., Suite #502
Doral, FL 33172
(305) 558-3300
www.yourheartflorida.com

33324
Cardiovascular Specialists of South Florida
10650 West State Rd. 84, Suite 104
Davie, FL 33324
(954) 382-1550

33410
Richard Price, MD
3365 Burns Road, Suite 207
Palm Beach Gardens, FL 33410
(561) 626-5606

33435
Anil Verma, MD
2580 S. Seacrest Blvd.
Boynton Beach, FL 33435
(561) 369-7865

33449
Cardiology Partners of the Palm Beaches
3347 State Rd 7, Suite 203
Wellington, FL 33449

(561) 793-6100

33462
Florida Cardiology Group, PA
110 JFK Drive, Suite 110
Atlantis, FL 33462
(561) 641-9541

33716
Millenium Health and Wellness
10033 Dr. Martin Luther King St., North, Ste 300
St. Petersburg, FL 33716
(727) 498-8988

34104
Evenhuis Cardiology & Internal Medicine
1351 Pine Street
Naples, FL 34104
(239) 262-5770

34239
Heart and Vascular Center of Sarasota
1851 Hawthorne Street
Sarasota, FL 34239
(941) 365-0433

34972
Treasure Coast Cardiology, PA
1713 Highway 441, North, Suite B
Okeechobee, FL 34972
(863) 467-9400

36301
Southeast Cardiology Clinic, Inc.

1150 Ross Clark Circle, SE
Dothan, AL 36301
(334) 712-2794

37923

Restoration Heart Care - Gregory Brewer, MD
314 Prosperity Drive
Knoxville, TN 37923
(865) 691-8011

39649

Cardiovascular Institute Of Mississippi
303 Marion Avenue
McComb, MS 39649
(601) 249-1348

42066

Jackson Purchase Medical Center
1099 Medical Center Circle
Mayfield, KY 42066
(270) 251-4100

42431

Heart Care Associates
44 McCoy Avenue, Suite 379, Box #9
Madisonville, KY 42431
(270) 821-0677

43606

EECP® Center of Northwest Ohio
3110 W. Central Avenue
Toledo, OH 43606
(419) 531-4235

www.heartfixer.com

43608

Toledo Cardiology Consultants
2409 Cherry Street, Suite 100
Toledo, OH 43608
(419) 251-3570

43615

Promedica Physician Group
2940 N. McCord Rd.
Toledo, OH 43615
(419) 842-3098

44805

Samaritan Hospital
1025 Center Street
Ashland, OH 44805
(419) 289-0491

47546

Memorial Hospital and Health Care Center
440 Scott Rolen Drive
Jasper, IN 47546
(812) 996-5702
(812) 996-0553

48073

Beaumont Health Center
4949 Coolidge Highway
Royal Oak, MI 48073
(248) 655-5750

48105

University of Michigan
24 Frank Lloyd Wright Dr.
Ann Arbor, MI 48105
(734) 998-9590

48236
St. John Hospital and Medical Center
Cardiac Rehab, 22151 Moross Rd, Suite 135, PB1
Detroit, MI 48236
(313) 343-4216
www.stjohn.org/eecp

48308
Rochester Medical Center
543 Main Street P. O. Box 82207
Rochester, MI 48308
(248) 656-3100

48336
Botsford Hospital
28050 Grand River Avenue
Farmington Hills, MI 48336
(248) 471-8087

48864
Lansing Cardiovascular Consultants
3413 Woods Edge Dr.
Okemos, MI 48864
(517) 349-3303

52803
Cardiovascular Medicine, PC
1236 E. Rusholme Street
Davenport, IA 52803

(563) 324-2992

54601

Mayo Clinic Health System, La Crosse
700 West Avenue South
La Crosse, WI 54601
(608) 526-3351

54601

Gundersen Lutheran
2101 Sims Place
La Crosse, WI 54601
(608) 775-4166

55407

Minneapolis Heart Institute
920 E. 28th Street, Suite 300
Minneapolis, MN 55407
(612) 863-7821

55415

Hennepin County Medical Center
701 Park Avenue-A5 Adabec 865A
Minneapolis, MN 55415
(612) 873-5569

55415

Hennepin County Medical Center
701 Park Avenue-A5 Adabec 865A
Minneapolis, MN 55415
(612) 873-5569

55426

Methodist Hospital

6500 Excelsior Blvd.
St. Louis Park, MN 55426
(952) 993-7014

55802
St. Luke's Hospital
1001 East Superior Street, Ste. L-201
Duluth, MN 55802
(218) 249-3057

55805
St. Mary's Duluth Clinic
407 E. Third Street
Duluth, MN 55805
(888) 253-0394

55905
Mayo Clinic Hospital
1216 2nd Street MB4-506
Rochester, MN 55905
(507) 255-8354

55987
Winona Health Services
855 Mankato Avenue
Winona, MN 55987
(507) 457-4419
www.winonahealth.org

56362
Paynesville Area Health System
200 First Street West
Paynesville, MN 56362
(320) 243-7708

56636

Deer River Healthcare Center
1002 Comstock Drive
Deer River, MN 56636
(218) 246-3034

57078

Avera Sacred Heart Hospital
501 Summit Street
Yankton, SD 57078
(605) 668-8000

57105

Avera McKennan Hospital
800 E. 21st Street
Sioux Falls, SD 57105
(605) 322-6500

57105

Sioux Valley Hospital
1305 W 18th Street Cath Lab
Sioux Falls, SD 57105
(605) 333-7266

57350

Huron Regional Medical Center
172 4th Street, SE
Huron, SD 57350
(605) 353-6237

59601

Universal Health Connection, Inc.
900 N. Montana Ave, Ste. B9

Helena, MT 59601
(406) 431-7332

62220
Cardiology Consultants
340 West Lincoln St.
Belleville, IL 62220
(618) 233-2969

62801
Naeem A. Khan, MD, SC
1050 M.L. King Drive, Suite 108
Centralia, IL 62801
(618) 532-8574

63028
Manzoor A. Tariq, MD
1071 Airport Road
Festus, MO 63028
(636) 937-7481

65109
Jefferson City Medical Group
1241 Stadium Blvd.
Jefferson City, MO 65109
(618) 532-8574

65804
Mercy Clinic Cardiology - Whiteside
2115 S. Fremont Avenue Suite 4300
Springfield, MO 65804
(417) 820-3911

71730

Heart Associates of South Arkansas
619 West Grove
El Dorado, AR 71730
(870) 863-6133

72019
Saline Heart Group, P.A.
1000 Highway 35 North, Suite 8
Benton, AR 72019
(501) 315-4008

72653
Cardiovascular Associates of N. Central AR
555 West 6th Street
Mountain Home, AR 72653
(870) 425-8288

75251
Trinity Heart Care
12230 Coit Rd
Dallas, TX 75251
(972) 490-9500
www.trinityheartcare.com

75701
Cardiovascular Associates of East TX, PA
1783 Troup Hwy.
Tyler, TX 75701
(903) 595-2283

75801
East Texas Physician's Alliance
112 East Oak
Palestine, TX 75801

(903) 723-8800

76102
Legacy Heart Care, Inc.
2500 West Freeway, Suite 200
Fort Worth, TX 76102
(817) 423-4400
www.legacyheartcare.com

76508
Scott & White Memorial Hospital
2401 South 31st Street
Temple, TX 76508
(254) 724-7437

77339
Cardiovascular Association, P.L.L.C
22999 US Highway 59
Kingwood, TX 77339
(281) 359-4888

77375
Northwest Heart Center
13406 Medical Complex Drive, Suite 110
Tomball, TX 77375
(281) 351-6250

77707
Cardiac Consultants
3345 Plaza 1- Drive, Suite E
Beaumont, TX 77707
(409) 838-2626

78240

Legacy Heart Care
2 Spurs Lane, Bldg 6 Suite 200
San Antonio, TX 78240
(210) 558-1800
www.legacyheartcare.com

78404

Cardiology Associates of Corpus Christi
1521 South Staples, #700
Corpus Christi, TX 78404
(361) 888-8271

78705

Legacy Heart Care - Austin
901 West 38th Street, Suite 403
Austin, TX 78705
(512) 419-1100
www.legacyheartcare.com

80120

South Denver Cardiology Associates
1000 So. Park Drive
Littleton, CO 80120
(303) 744-1065

81601

Valley View Hospital
1906 Blake Avenue
Glenwood Springs, CO 81601
(970) 384-7320

83301

St. Luke's Cardiology Clinic (EECP)
775 Pole Line Road West, Suite 112

Twin Falls, ID 83301
(208) 814-8222

85282
Legacy Heart Care
4515 S. McClintock Dr., Suite 120
Tempe, AZ 85282
(480) 704-3700
www.legacyheartcare.com

85381
Cardiac Solutions - Peoria
13128 N. 94th Drive #100
Peoria, AZ 85381
(623) 876-8816

85701
Carondelet Heart and Vascular Imaging at St.Vincent's
6567 E. Carondelet Drive, Ste 225
Tucson, AZ 85710
(520) 873-6612

85901
Summit Healthcare - Cardiovascular Services
5300 S. Sutter Dr. Suite 1
Show Low, AZ 85901
(928) 527-4375

86001
Mountain Heart
2000 S. Thompson St.
Flagstaff, AZ 86001
(303) 744-1065

86403

Lakeside Heart & Vascular Center
2082 Mesquite Ave., Ste. 100A
Lake Havasu City, AZ 86403
(928) 453-2727
www.lakesideheart.com

86409

Heart Institute of North Arizona
1753 Airway Avenue, Suite B
Kingman, AZ 86409
(928) 692-6200

88011

Southwest Cardiovascular Center
1255 S. Telshor Blvd.
Las Cruces, NM 88011
(575) 522-0300

89119

Nevada Heart and Vascular Center, LLC
4725 S. Burnham Ave., Suite #100
Las Vegas, NV 89119
(702) 240-8273

89128

Nevada Heart and Vascular Center, LLC
7455 West Washington Ave, Suite 300
Las Vegas, NV 89128
(702) 240-8273

89502

Renown Institute for Heart

1500 E 2nd, Ste. #400
Reno, NV 89502
(775) 982-4780

89511
Dr. David Edwards, M.D.
615 Sierra Rosa Dr.
Reno, NV 89511
(775) 828-4055

90025
Global Cardio Care, Inc.
11860 Wilshire Blvd.
Los Angeles, CA 90025
(310) 473-3030
www.globalcardiocare.com

90033
East LA Cardiology Medical Group
1701 East Cesar E. Chavez Ave, Ste. 125
Los Angeles, CA 90033
(323) 441-1122

90033
Pure Heart EECP
1701 E Caesar Chavez Blvd
Los Angeles, CA 90033
(818) 395-8561

90048
Cedar Sinai Medical Center
127 South San Vincente Blvd.
Los Angeles, CA 90048
(310) 428-3838

90255

Rumi Lakha, DO
7136 Pacific Blvd #220
Huntington Park, CA 90255
(323) 588-5467

90301

Global Cardio Care, Inc.
633 Aerick Street, Suite 101
Inglewood, CA 90301
(310) 412-8181
www.globalcardiocare.com

91007

Diagnostic Heart Center
624 W. Duarte Road, Suite 207
Arcadia, CA 91007
(626) 446-5800

91203

Glendale Heart Institute Medical Group, Inc.
435 Arden Avenue, Suite 410
Glendale, CA 91203
(818) 242-4191

91204

Southern California Cardiovascular Consultants
1510 South Central Avenue
Glendale , CA 91204
(818) 242-8816

91204

California Cardiac Institute
710 S. Central Avenue, Suite 200
Glendale, CA 91204
(818) 247-0346

94520
Cardiac Heart Recirculation Centers, Inc.
2270 Bacon Street
Concord, CA 94520
(925) 938-5400

94535
David Grant USAF Medical Center
101 Bodin Circle
Travis AFB, CA 94535
(707) 423-3277

95076
Brennon Medical Group
30 Brenan Street
Watsonville, CA 95076
(831) 768-0220

95112
Ngai Nguyen, MD
696 East Santa Clara Street, Suite 108
San Jose, CA 95112
(408) 971-8441

95403
Northern California Medical Associates
3536 Mendocino Ave. Suite 200
Santa Rosa, CA 95403
(707) 573-6166

95667

Marshall Medical Center
1100 Marshall Way
Placerville, CA 95667
(530) 626-2770
www.marshallmedical.org

95817

UC Davis Medical Center
4860 Y Street
Sacramento, CA 95817
(916) 734-3761

96093

Trinity Alps Medical Group
500 Trinity Lakes Blvd.
Weaverville, CA 96093
(530) 623-6777

96734

Windward Vein, Heart, and Medispa
25 Maluniu Ave Suite #202
Kailua, HI 96734
808-281-2441

96740

Island Heart Care
75-167 Hualalai Rd # 100
 Kailua-Kona, HI 96740
(808) 769-5225

96743

Island Heart Care
64-1035 Mamalahoa Highway, Suite J
Kamuela, HI 96743
(808) 885-4507

97220
Integrated Medicine Group
163 Northeast 102nd Avenue, Building 5
Portland, OR 97220
(503) 257-3327

97504
Asante Health System - Rogue Valley Medical Center
2825 E. Barnett Rd.
Medford , OR 97504
(541) 789-5049

98052
David S. Buscher, MD
8195 166th Avenue NE
Redmond, WA 98052
(425) 284-1586

98632
St. John's Medical Center
1615 Delaware Street
Longview, WA 98632
(360) 414-7384

99508
Alaska Regional Community Health Clinic
3701 Mountain View Dr
Anchorage, AK 99508

(907) 770-1430

ABOUT THE AUTHOR

Survivor of eleven heart attacks before doctors discovered their underlying cause, Robert Rister has written dozens of books and given thousands of presentations on medical and science topics.